MW01256201

Dietary Supplements

Dietary Supplements

B. Bryan Haycock and Amy A. Sunderman

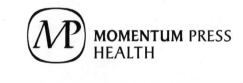

MOMENTUM PRESS HEALTH

MOMENTUM PRESS, LLC, NEW YORK

Dietary Supplements

Copyright © Momentum Press, LLC, 2016.

All rights reserved. No part of this publication may be reproduced, stored in a retrieval system, or transmitted in any form or by any means—electronic, mechanical, photocopy, recording, or any other except for brief quotations, not to exceed 400 words, without the prior permission of the publisher.

First published in 2016 by
Momentum Press, LLC
222 East 46th Street, New York, NY 10017
www.momentumpress.net

ISBN-13: 978-1-60650-755-1 (paperback)
ISBN-13: 978-1-60650-756-8 (e-book)

Momentum Press Nutrition and Dietetics Practice Collection

Cover and interior design by Exeter Premedia Services Private Ltd., Chennai, India

First edition: 2016

10 9 8 7 6 5 4 3 2 1

Printed in the United States of America.

Abstract

The purpose of this book is to provide an overview of dietary supplements including their definition according to the Dietary Supplement Health and Education Act, how they are manufactured and regulated, what forms they are sold in, and what the most popular products are. In discussing the most popular products people use, an effort is made to provide information on the background or origin of each ingredient. In addition, the potential mechanism of action and the clinical evidence that may exist demonstrating the efficacy or lack thereof is reviewed.

This book is important given the fact that the sale and use of dietary supplements is a controversial issue. The media frequently broadcasts negative stories about the dietary supplement industry and its products and elicit the testimonies of individuals without expertise in the industry, or the science behind dietary supplements. Furthermore, the supplement industry is rife with unscrupulous fly-by-night companies that make false and misleading claims about their products, further damaging the perception of the industry. If that were all there was to the story, there would be no need for this book. On the contrary, epidemiological data demonstrates that the proper use of dietary supplements could save thousands of lives and billions of dollars in health care costs. This book is an attempt to contribute an objective perspective on the matter.

Keywords

caffeine, coenzyme Q10, dietary supplement, DSHEA, fiber, glucosamine, microbiome, mineral, omega-3, prebiotic, probiotic, resolving, vitamin, vitamin D, weight loss

Contents

Acknowledgments

I wish to personally thank the following people who without their contributions and support this book would not have been written. All the people at Momentum Press and especially executive editor Peggy Williams and series editor Katie Ferraro for their guidance and patience throughout the writing process. Douglas "Duffy" MacKay for his generous help and contributions to the regulatory history section of this book. Luke Bucci for serving as both my mentor and role model in the dietary supplement industry. Wayne Askew without whose faith and generosity towards me I would not be where I am today. My friend, colleague, and coauthor Amy A. Sunderman without whose contributions writing this book would not have been possible. Finally, my wife and family who have supported me, believed in me, and enabled me to accomplish so much and meet the many obligations I seem to bring upon myself.

CHAPTER 1

Introduction

Overview

This chapter provides an overview of dietary supplements including their definition according to the Dietary Supplement Health and Education Act (DSHEA). How each class of dietary supplement is manufactured, what dosage forms they are sold in, and what coating or release technology might be applied to the products are discussed. A brief history of the dietary supplement industry regulation is also given. Landmark episodes in the history of dietary supplements regulation are discussed including the time before regulation. It is intended that enough depth should be provided to satisfy the layperson's curiosity about such aspects of dietary supplements without going into technical details requiring any special background knowledge or education to understand.

What Are Dietary Supplements?

In the simplest terms, dietary supplements are nutritional products taken by people for any number of reasons, but generally they are products that just do something good for their health. From a legal standpoint, dietary supplements have a more specific definition. The DSHEA of 1994 defined a dietary supplement in the following terms.

A product (other than tobacco) intended to supplement the diet and that bears or contains one or more of the following dietary ingredients:

- Vitamins
- Minerals
- Herbs and botanicals
- Herbal and botanical extracts
- Animal extracts

- Amino acids
- Proteins
- Concentrates, metabolites, constituents
- Teas
- Other ingredients

See Table 1.1 for a list giving the definition for each ingredient category. In addition, these products must be designed for ingestion in

Table 1.1 Categories and definitions of dietary supplement ingredients

Substance	Definition
Vitamins	Products that are organic (carbon-containing) nutrients that are essential in small quantities for normal metabolism, growth, and well-being. They must be obtained through the diet because they are either not synthesized in the body or not synthesized in adequate amounts
Minerals	Products that are chemical elements in their inorganic forms. "Minerals" are those that are required in amounts greater than 100 mg/day, and "trace minerals" are those required in lesser amounts
Herbs and botanicals	Herbal or botanical products prepared by means other than extraction (i.e., dried, crushed, and encapsulated). These may include teas in addition to other product forms. The term herbal refers to the leaves and stems of the plant while botanical refers to these parts in addition to roots, seeds, and fruits
Herbal and botanical extracts	Products that are extracts obtained from any part of a plant
Animal extracts	Products that are extracts obtained from animal parts (e.g., tissues and glands)
Amino acids	Products that contain an amino group and an acidic function
Proteins	Products with the complete set of amino acids to make up proteins
Concentrates, metabolites, constituents	Products that are concentrated, are broken down into individual components, or are parts of other products
Teas	Products containing herbals, botanicals, or other dietary supplements that are infused in water. Basic tea products have a standard of identity as a food product; however, many products are a combination of tea and dietary supplements
Other	All other products meeting the criteria of dietary supplements that cannot be classified into the categories mentioned here. They include, for example, bee pollen, propolis, and royal jelly; coenzyme Q10; spirulina and other algae; and nucleic acids

pill, capsule, tablet, or liquid form; must not be represented as a food or sole item of a meal or diet; and must be labeled as a "dietary supplement."

How Dietary Supplements Are Manufactured

Dietary supplements include a wide variety of nutritional compounds and edible substances. Even the definition of a dietary supplement defined by DSHEA, though brief, includes many possible different substances and sources. The manufacture of large quantities of individual nutrients required to meet demand is accomplished through a number of means—from simple drying and crushing of herbs to multistep chemical synthesis. We discuss here each of the major methods of manufacturing dietary supplements beginning with vitamins.

Vitamins

Vitamins are organic compounds consumed in the diet in small quantities. An organic compound qualifies as a vitamin if its absence from the diet produces overt symptoms of deficiency. These symptoms range from the troublesome, such as itchy skin, to life threatening ones. The symptoms indicate that the compound cannot be synthesized in the body, and thus it is essential that it be consumed in adequate amounts as a supplement to maintain health or allow proper development. There are 13 nutrients classified as vitamins: vitamins B1, B2, B3, B6, B12, C, A, D, E, K, biotin, folic acid, and pantothenic acid. Vitamins are categorized according to their solubility in water or fat. Vitamins B1, B2, B3, B6, B12, C, biotin, folic acid, and pantothenic acid are water-soluble. Vitamins A, D, E, and K are fat-soluble. There are three large-scale manufacturing methods used to produce vitamins for commercial use: synthesis, fermentation, and extraction (Muth et al. 1999).

Chemical Synthesis

The production of vitamins by chemical synthesis involves basic chemicals reacting together to produce the desired compound. Historically speaking, when a vitamin was discovered and a source identified, the chemical structure was determined, and then its synthesis was worked out on a small scale. Then it was just a matter of scaling up to a commercial scale. The majority of vitamins are still produced in this manner. Vitamin E can be synthesized but it can also be extracted from vegetable oil. Vitamin B12 is the only vitamin that is not produced by chemical synthesis, and this is due to its molecular complexity.

Fermentation

Fermentation is the next most common manufacturing process for vitamins; even so, only Vitamin B12 is produced this way. Humans do not produce the necessary enzymes to make vitamin B12; bacteria however do. For this reason, Vitamin B12 is manufactured using bacteria. Fermentation involves growing bacteria in large tanks. The bacteria are fed and cultured in a way that maximizes production of the desired end product, in this case vitamin B12. When mature, the bacteria are separated from the growth medium, dried, and lysed. Then the desired compound is isolated from the cellular mass. Isolation often requires the use of solvents.

Extraction

After the discovery of vitamins, they were isolated by extraction from natural sources. For example, vitamin B6 was isolated from rice, vitamin B2 from eggs, and vitamin B12, niacin, and biotin from liver. Vitamins A and D were isolated from cod liver oil, vitamin E from wheat germ oil, and vitamin K from alfalfa. Today, however, because of the large demand, it is not feasible to extract vitamins from natural sources, the one exception being Vitamin E, which is extracted from vegetable oil.

Minerals

Like vitamins, minerals are required in the diet for health and proper development. Unlike vitamins, however, minerals are inorganic substances. Minerals required in quantities greater than 100 mg/day are just called minerals, while those required in quantities less than 100 mg/day are called trace minerals or sometimes trace elements. Dietary minerals are produced by extracting them from rock and soil. In addition to rock and soil, they often come from places where mineral deposits are highly concentrated, such as around small seas or terminal lakes. Even supplements that claim to contain "plant minerals" may actually come from sedimentary rock (Muth et al. 1999). Some products may claim that they contain a mineral "chelate." A chelate is an ionic compound, usually organic, that forms a bond with metal. In dietary supplements, it is usually an amino acid of some sort. Evidence that chelating a mineral improves its safety or bioavailability is lacking. Finally, mineral supplements are sometimes sold as colloidal minerals. A colloidal mineral is one that has been ground into extremely fine particles that are able to stay suspended in a liquid without settling.

Herbs, Algae, and Herbal Extracts

Herbs used in dietary supplements come from all over the world. Most are grown on farms. Herbal dietary supplements can be purchased as a straight herb or as an herbal extract. To produce a straight herbal product, the herb is grown, cultivated, harvested, and then dried before processing for shipment and manufacture. Processing involves cleaning the plant material to remove any dirt, bugs, or foreign bodies picked up during harvesting. In many instances, only the leaf, stem, or root is used so the material must be sifted, sorted, and separated. Once the desired part of the herb has been separated, the particle size must be reduced to a uniform size for manufacturing into tablets and capsules. This can be done by shredding, crushing, grinding, or milling the material.

Although most herbs and botanical ingredients are farmed, some are collected from the wild. In such cases sustainability becomes an important issue to ensure future supply as well as to preserve the natural ecosystems. A survey of the herbal trade market found that existing industry practice often promotes poor management of species and few benefits for local communities, and that many companies remain distant from and unaware of the conditions under which the raw materials are sourced. However, opportunities exist to create a change as more and more industries that make dietary supplements as well as other industries that use botanical ingredients take responsibility for sustainable sourcing of raw materials (Laird, Pierce, and Schmitt 2005).

Although not technically an herb, algae are a single-celled plant species consumed as a dietary supplement. Algae for human consumption are produced in two basic ways: harvesting it from open ponds and using closed system photobioreactors. Each system has its advantages and disadvantages.

Open ponds are shallow, manmade pools that are typically built in such a way that paddle wheels or other mechanisms can keep the water in slow and constant motion. For algae to flourish in open ponds, constant addition of nutrients and carbon dioxide is required. While open ponds are relatively simple and inexpensive systems, they do have some drawbacks, such as space limitations, unpredictable weather, variable light utilization, evaporation, and pond contamination, all of which reduce yields.

A closed system photobioreactor consists of rows of connected glass or plastic tubes with diameters ranging between 5 and 30 cm. Closed systems allow for more control of ideal growing conditions by providing accurate monitoring of nutrients, pH, oxygen, and carbon dioxide levels to produce higher and more consistent yields. Photobioreactors can be built outdoors to utilize natural sunlight, or they can be indoors and use fiber optic lights. Fiber optic lights allow the lighting system to be placed within the water-filled tubes without transmitting electricity or heat. The greatest control of yields comes from the use of artificial lights with some producers even controlling the UV spectrum used for growth. Closed systems also enable growers to easily collect and move algae. The obvious drawback to these types of systems is the cost.

In addition to algae that is grown for consumption, algae that is used to produce other ingredients such as omega-3 fatty acids and the carotenoid astaxanthin is grown with these two systems.

Herbal Extracts

Herbal extracts are chemicals extracted from plant material by means of a solvent. There are a number of methods used to produce extracts including organic solvents extraction, supercritical gas extraction, and steam distillation (Gil-Chávez et al. 2013; Muth et al. 1999).

Organic Solvent Extraction

Solvent extraction works by enabling the separation of chemicals based on their solubility in different solvents. Most solvents used for the production of herbal extracts are volatile organic compounds such as hexane, ether, chloroform, acetonitrile, benzene, and ethanol. These are commonly used in different ratios with water (Gil-Chávez et al. 2013).

Before a substance can be extracted with a solvent, the cells of the plant material must be lysed, and this can be done by crushing, grinding, or milling. Ultrasound techniques are sometimes used to disintegrate intact cells exposing the intracellular compartments to the solvent. After the application of the solvent, the desired chemical will dissolve into the solvent, producing a solution called the "miscella." The miscella is then drained from the plant material. The miscella will usually have other undesirable compounds in it; so further purification steps are necessary. This might involve decanting, filtration, sedimentation, centrifuging, heating, adsorption, precipitation, or ion exchange filtration of the miscella (Muth et al. 1999). At this point, the desired compound and residual solvent are still in a liquid solution and in order to obtain the pure compound, the solvent must be removed. Depending on the resilience of the compound, drying can be done by vacuum freeze dryers, cabinet vacuum dryers, drum or belt dryers, microwave ovens, or atomizers. Because of potential toxicity of some solvents, it is important that all residual traces of the solvent be removed in the drying process.

Steam Distillation

Steam distillation is another method for extracting active ingredients from herbal plant material. The process involves injecting steam through a fluid mixture of the raw plant material. The vapor mixture is cooled, condensed, and drained yielding a liquid with a layer of oil on top and a lower layer of water distillate. The oil is called the essential oil of that particular herb. The remaining water contains the desired compound that must then be purified and dried.

At this point, it is worth mentioning that teas are also considered dietary supplements according to the DSHEA. As such, tea would fall into the category of a water extract for immediate use.

Supercritical Fluid Extraction

Supercritical fluid extraction (sometimes called supercritical gas extraction) is a method by which a gas is brought to a temperature and pressure at which it remains in a gaseous state but has the density of a fluid. It is in this "supercritical" state that it is used as a solvent. For dietary supplements, several gases can be used but carbon dioxide is the gas of choice because it is nontoxic and does not harm the environment. For this process, the raw material is placed in a container called an extractor vessel, which has temperature and pressure controllers to maintain the desired conditions. The gas dissolves the desired compounds within the plant material and then passes into a separating chamber where both pressure and temperature are lower. Once the fluid and the dissolved compounds are transported to separators, the products are collected through a valve at the bottom of the separator tank. This process produces a solvent-free extract.

Amino Acids

Amino acids are organic compounds containing both an amine group and a carboxylic acid functional group. Amino acids are frequently referred to as the building blocks of protein because proteins consist of chains of amino acids. When it comes to the manufacture of amino acids, the important thing to know is that amino acids are "chiral" compounds. This means that they exist in two forms or enantiomers that are mirror images of one another. Chiral enantiomers are like your right and left hands; they are the same but are mirror images of each other. The two chiral forms are designated as L and D. Humans can only use the L form of amino acids for protein synthesis. The D form amino acids, such as d-aspartate, can be found in the body but cannot be incorporated into proteins, and they are not essential in the diet. The amino acids used in dietary supplements are the L form and are labeled L-leucine, and L-arginine, for example.

You can synthesize amino acids from basic chemicals for use as dietary supplements. This produces a 50–50 mix of the L form and D form. This means you must divide whatever yield you get in half, because only the L form can be used. The primary way of producing amino acids is by fermentation. Both bacteria and yeast are able to produce amino acids efficiently with a high yield, and because bacteria and yeast are living organisms, they produce pure L form amino acids. The process of fermentation is similar to what has been described earlier for vitamins.

Protein Powders

Protein powders come in three forms, concentrate, isolate, and hydrolysate. Whey protein concentrate, for example, is made by passing the liquid whey, a byproduct of processed cheese, through pasteurization, a separator, and then ultrafiltration and diafiltration. Ultrafiltration and diafiltration are processes that use semipermeable membranes to sequentially filter nonprotein components of raw whey until the desired concentration of protein is achieved. The resulting protein-rich liquid is then dried through spray drying, which removes almost all of the water. Whey concentrate contains between 65 to 80 percent protein as well as some residual lactose, fat, and minerals. Protein isolates, such as whey isolate, are produced in the same way but with an extra filtration step to remove any remaining lactose, fat, and minerals, thus bringing the protein concentration up to 90 percent.

Some protein powders and baby formulas contain protein hydrolysates. Protein hydrolysates are peptides and amino acids derived from protein isolates by exposing them to enzymes or acids. The most commonly used enzymes for protein hydrolysates are pancreatin, trypsin, pepsin, papain, bromelain, and bacterial and fungal proteases. The hydrolysis of proteins can be achieved by a single enzymatic step or a sequential enzyme hydrolysis using multiple enzymes (Pasupuleti and Braun 2010). The result is a powder that is very bitter to taste and, therefore, can only be used in small amounts in dietary protein supplements.

Animal Products

Some dietary supplements contain animal tissue or extracts from tissues or glands. Some of these products are manufactured by solvent extraction, while others are composed of intact dehydrated tissue. For example, chondroitin sulfate, a popular clinically studied dietary supplement used to promote joint health, is extracted mainly from cow and pig cartilage. There are also supplements as well as pharmaceutical products made by freeze-drying animal glands such as the thyroid and pituitary glands. Freeze-dried animal glands have residual hormones within them, and are believed to retain hormonal action when taken orally.

Bees, though technically not animals, are also a source of some dietary supplements. Three products in particular are used as dietary supplements: propolis, bee pollen, and royal jelly. Propolis is a substance made by bees that consist of plant resins mixed with wax. Bees use it as a sort of environmental barrier, coating the inside of the hive with a thin layer of propolis. It is thought to provide some antimicrobial protection for the bees (Simone-Finstrom and Spivak 2012). Propolis can be collected by scraping it from the interior of the beehive. Propolis production can be induced by placing a plastic mesh barrier within the hive creating a temporary partition. The bees will then cover the plastic mesh with propolis in an attempt to seal off the hive. The mesh can then be removed, and the propolis scraped off. An average size hive can produce about 200 g of propolis per year.

Bee pollen can also be collected. Bees collect pollen from flowers and bring it back to the hive where it is combined with nectar to feed the colony and produce honey. Screens can be placed at the entrance of a hive forcing the bees to squeeze through as they enter. As they squeeze through the holes in the screen, a small amount of pollen is scraped off the bee and falls into a collector tray below. As much as 2 to 3 kg can be collected in this manner without causing a shortage of pollen for the hive (Muth et al. 1999).

Royal jelly is a food produced by nursing bees to feed the larvae that are to become queen bees. To collect it, special movable comb hives are used. Queen cells, which are wax chambers that contain queen bee larvae, are placed in a hive causing the bees to start producing royal jelly. After the cell containing the larvae has been filled with royal jelly, the larvae is removed so the jelly can be collected. Each cell contains approximately 200 mg of royal jelly. Royal jelly is perishable and must be refrigerated or frozen after it is collected.

Other Miscellaneous Ingredients

The production methods of common types of dietary ingredients have been discussed here. A variety of other ingredients can also be found in products falling under the category of "constituents, metabolites, and concentrates" that were not mentioned specifically, but generally involve the same kind of manufacturing processes.

Dietary Supplements Come in Many Different Forms

Pertinent to our discussion of the manufacture of raw materials used in dietary supplements are finished dosage forms. The finished dosage form relates to the form of the product that is intended for use by the consumer. For dietary supplements, this includes pills, capsules, powders, and liquids. Table 1.2 contains the most common dosage forms of dietary supplements (Food and Drug Administration [FDA] 2009).

Table 1.2 Common dosage forms of dietary supplements

Dosage form	Description
Tablet	A dosage form of dry ingredients compressed into a pill. Tablets can be any shape and size conducive to swallowing. Tablets may contain active ingredients blended uniformly throughout or separated into different layers within the tablet.
Chewable tablet	A tablet that is intended to be chewed before swallowing. Chewable tablets are made using lower compression forces and with additional excipients to allow the tablet to dissolve in the mouth as it is chewed. Chewable tablets are convenient for individuals who have difficulty swallowing pills.
Capsule	A dosage form consisting of a shell and a filling. The shell is composed of two halves that fit together that is sometimes sealed with a band. Capsule shells may be made from gelatin, starch, or cellulose, or other suitable materials and filled with dry or liquid ingredients.

(Continued)

Table 1.2 Common dosage forms of dietary supplements   **(Continued)**

Dosage form	Description
Softgel	A softgel is a type of soft capsule filled with liquid ingredients. The shell consists of gelatin, water, and a plasticizer such as glycerin or sorbitol. Softgels can be made into various shapes and sizes conducive to swallowing.
Powder	Powders may be coarse or fine and are often agglomerated to enhance dissolution when stirred into a liquid. Powders are used when large serving sizes are required.
Liquid or emulsion	Active ingredients can be dissolved or blended into any liquid approved for human consumption. An emulsion is a two-component mixture comprised of at least two immiscible liquids, one of which is dispersed as droplets (normally oil) within the other liquid (normally water), and stabilized with one or more emulsifying agents. Limitations are placed on the volume of liquid per serving to be classified as a dietary supplement and not a beverage.
Effervescent	An active ingredient in a dry mixture usually combined with sodium bicarbonate, citric acid, and tartaric acid, which when placed in water, releases carbon dioxide gas resulting in effervescence. Dosage form may be a powder or tablet intended to be dissolved in water before consuming.
Chew	A chew is an extruded semisolid dosage form meant to be chewed before swallowing. Chews are convenient for individuals who have difficulty swallowing pills.
Gummy	A gummy is a gelatin-based soft chewable candy containing active ingredients. Gummies are convenient for individuals who have difficulty swallowing pills.
Lozenge	A hard candy-like dosage form that is intended to dissolve or disintegrate slowly in the mouth.
Strip	A strip is a thin film-like dry dosage form that is intended to be placed on the tongue and allowed to dissolve in the mouth. Strips are physically limited in the amount of active ingredient they can contain.

Coatings and Release Technologies

Not only do dietary supplements come in multiple dosage forms but they can also have different coatings and dissolution or release characteristics. Examples include enteric coating, microencapsulation, delayed release, and extended release technologies.

Enteric coating is the process of coating a tablet or capsule with an edible polymer that allows transit through the stomach before the active ingredient is released. Enteric refers to the small intestine. It serves to protect the active ingredient from the acidic environment of the stomach. Likewise, it can be used to protect the lining of the stomach from ingredients that can irritate the stomach. Normally the enteric coating is pH sensitive, remaining intact in acidic pH then dissolving at a more basic pH.

Delayed release is a term used to describe a product that does not dissolve in the stomach. This can be accomplished by the use of enteric coating or by the use of binders that help to keep the tablet intact for a given amount of time after ingestion. Delayed release is a characteristic of many enteric coated dosage forms.

Sustained release is a term used to describe the rate at which an active ingredient is released from the tablet or capsule. Like delayed release dosage forms, sustained release forms generally utilize binders that slowly disintegrate over time allowing a slow and sustained release of the active as it travels through the digestive tract. This is beneficial when the active ingredient has a short half-life.

Microencapsulation is a process of encapsulating microscopic particles of dry or liquid ingredients. Various technologies can be used to first disperse the active ingredients into microscopic size particles and then enveloping those particles in a thin polymer coating. This method can be used to turn oils into powders. Microencapsulation is useful when an active ingredient is unstable or has an unpleasant flavor or smell. Once a raw material has been microencapsulated, it can be incorporated into almost any dosage form.

Dietary Supplement Regulation

Brief History of Regulation Leading to the DSHEA

In the United States, dietary supplements are regulated by a comprehensive set of laws and regulations set forth in the Federal Food, Drug, and Cosmetic Act (FDCA) of 1938, and later amended by the DSHEA of 1994 (See Table 1.3 for a chronology of the legislative acts associated with dietary supplements). This set of legislations gives the FDA jurisdiction over product safety, manufacturing, and labeling. Advertising of dietary supplements is overseen by the Federal Trade Commission (FTC), also established in 1938 by the Wheeler–Lea Act. Together, the FDA and FTC provide broad federal oversight of the dietary supplement industry as a whole.

Today, the statutes and regulations governing the dietary supplement industry are quite comprehensive, regulating everything from manufacturing to the wording used to market dietary supplements. This was not always the case, however, and we must look back well over a century to see where the first federal regulatory efforts began and why.

The Federal Food and Drugs Act of 1906, better known as the Wiley Act, was the first federal act passed to regulate food and drug production and transport. It prohibited the manufacture of any food or drug that was adulterated or misbranded. It also prohibited the transport of adulterated, misbranded, or otherwise unlawful foods or drugs across state lines or their importation from another country.

At the time, dietary supplements were yet to be conceived of as such, but there were folk remedies and "patent medicines," which were the ancestors of both modern day drugs and dietary supplements. These concoctions and patent medicines, or nostrums as they were called, were sold as remedies for virtually any ailment. Much of the folk medicine was based on the idea that nature or God has provided remedies for common ailments of humanity in the fauna and flora of the geographical area where those ailments are most likely to occur (Young 1972). The patent medicines were called so because they were remedies that had received patents in Europe before being exported to the colonies of the United States. The many herbs, herbal extracts, glandular extracts, and drugs found in these remedies and patent medicines are too numerous to elaborate on here, but to give you an idea of the scene, it was not uncommon to find any number of opiates, cocaine, and even neurological poisons in these products. The product labels were not required to list the ingredients or warnings of any kind. Moreover, this had been going on for over a century before formal legislation was proposed.

In 1905, an American writer named Samuel Hopkins Adams wrote a series of 11 articles for Collier's Weekly entitled "The Great American Fraud" (Adams 1911; Fee 2010). Adams exposed many of the false claims made by the purveyors of patent medicines, bringing to the public's attention the many adverse and, in some cases, fatal events resulting from the use of such products. The articles were very influential and contributed in part to the passage of the 1906 Pure Food and Drug Act (PFDA).

In 1911, the Supreme Court ruled that the prohibition of falsifications referred only to the ingredients of the medicine and not its claims of efficacy. This meant that companies were again free to make false claims about their products. This inspired Adams to write another series of articles in Collier's Weekly exposing the false and misleading advertising that companies were using to sell their products. Both series of articles were reprinted as a book in 1911 (Adams 1911).

We now jump to 1938 and the passage of the FDCA. The FDCA essentially replaced the Federal Food and Drugs Act of 1906. In the intervening years between 1906 and 1938, the science of human nutrition and the role of "essential" nutrients progressed, and by the 1920s and 1930s, the public at large had become aware of the concept and importance of vitamins.

Cod liver oil was marketed in 1920 to supply extra Vitamin D and Vitamin A (Hutt 2005). This is perhaps the first food supplement marketed as a dietary supplement. Later in 1934, a true vitamin and mineral supplement was produced and marketed by the Nutrilite Company (Wallace and MacKay 2013). It was crude by today's standards, made simply by drying and compressing vegetable and fruit juice concentrates into a tablet, but it was by definition a true dietary supplement product.

The FDCA of 1938 recognized that foods could be and were being marketed using claims about their nutritional value, even making what would be considered structure function claims to describe the benefits of consuming it. At the same time, the FDA used the drug provisions of the law to gain greater control and reclassify dietary supplements as drugs based on their label claims. With this act, the FDA was also granted authority to inspect the manufacturing facilities of food, drug, and cosmetic companies. This same year, an amendment was made to the FTC Act to grant FTC oversight of the advertising for FDA-regulated products (except prescription drugs). Today the FTC is the primary enforcer of laws protecting the public against false and misleading claims made by dietary supplement marketers.

In 1941, the FDA added language to specifically address food products marketed with a "special dietary use" label (Porter and Earl 1990). Food products with a special dietary use were defined as used for supplying particular dietary needs that exist by reason of a physical, physiological, pathological, or other conditions, including but not limited to the conditions of disease, convalescence, pregnancy, lactation, allergic hypersensitivity to food, underweight, and overweight. All products falling into this category, which obviously included dietary supplements, were required to have labeling declaring the name, quantity, and percent Minimum Daily Requirement of each added nutrient (6 Fed. Reg. 5921 [Nov. 22, 1941]). This part of the code of regulations remains unchanged to this day.

The next significant legislative act affecting dietary supplements happened in 1976 with the passage of the Proxmire Amendments (Public Law 94-278). Going back for a moment to events leading up to the Proxmire Amendments in the 1960s and early 1970s, the FDA attempted to limit the allowable formulations and potency of vitamin and mineral supplements. In 1962, the agency published a proposed notice that "only those nutrients recognized by 'competent authorities' as essential and of significant human value could be offered for sale" (27 Fed. Reg. 5815, 5817 [June 20, 1962]) (Scarbrough 2004 Third Year Paper). The FDA proposed to limit the potency of vitamins and minerals to 150 percent of the reference values. If a dietary supplement exceeded 150 percent of the reference value with one or more vitamins or minerals, the product would be classified as a drug. In addition to the potency of vitamins and minerals, the agency attempted to limit the number and types of combinations of vitamins and minerals that could be sold by issuing a regulation in 1973 that established a Standard of Identity for vitamin and mineral supplements (38 FR 20,730, 20732 [August 2, 1973]) (Wallace and MacKay 2013). Arriving full circle, in 1976 in response to pressure from the public and dietary supplement industry, Congress passed the Proxmire Amendments (1976 Proxmire Amendment, 21 USC §350 [April 22, 1976]). These amendments prevented FDA from limiting the formulations and potency of vitamins and minerals in nutritional supplements and nullified the agency's authority to classify a vitamin or mineral product as a drug based solely on its potency. The Proxmire Amendments reinstated the original language of FDCA classifying drugs as, "intended for use in the diagnosis, cure, mitigation, treatment, or prevention of disease in man or other animals." (52 Stat 1040 [1938], 21 USC §301 et seq.). This would not be the last time the FDA attempted to limit the formulation of dietary supplements and reclassify them as drugs.

Some 20 years after the proposals put forth in 1973, the FDA issued an advanced notice of proposed rulemaking (ANPR). In this ANPR, the agency again attempted to restrict the potency of vitamins and minerals. It also declared that amino acids are food additives and were not legal in dietary supplements, and that herbal products are inherently therapeutic and should not be sold as dietary supplements. (58 FR 33690 [June 18, 1993]). Then in 1994, seeing that without some action on the part of Congress, the dietary supplement industry was in danger of excessive regulation, Senators Orrin Hatch and Tom Harkin drafted the DSHEA.

The Dietary Supplement Health and Education Act

According to U.S. Government Accountability Office, there were about 4,000 dietary supplement products on the market in 1994 when DSHEA was enacted (U.S. Government Accountability Office, 2009 GAO report—FDA should take further actions to improve oversight and consumer understanding, GAO-09-250). That number has grown significantly since then, likely closer to 40,000 today. With so many products available to consumers, it became evident that a more proactive regulatory framework was needed. DSHEA was enacted for this purpose and was intended to: (1) establish a new framework for assuring safety, (2) outline guidelines for literature displayed where supplements are sold, (3) provide for use claims and nutritional support statements, (4) require ingredient and nutrition labeling, (5) grant FDA the authority to establish good manufacturing practice (GMP) regulations, and (6) form an executive level Commission on Dietary Supplement Labels and an Office of Dietary Supplements (ODS) within the National Institutes of Health (NIH).

Prior to DSHEA, nutritional supplements were regulated primarily as food products. DSHEA provides an unambiguous definition of a dietary supplement and dictates when a product is to be regulated as a food or as a dietary supplement. DSHEA defines a dietary supplement as:

Any product that:

- is intended to supplement the diet and that bears or contains one or more of the following dietary ingredients: a vitamin, a mineral, an herb (other than tobacco) or other botanical, an amino acid (a dietary substance for use by man to supplement the diet by increasing the total daily intake), or a concentrate, metabolite, constituent, extract, or combinations of these ingredients;
- is intended for ingestion in pill, capsule, tablet, or liquid form;
- is not represented for use as a conventional food or as the sole item of a meal or diet;
- is labeled as a "dietary supplement"; and
- includes products such as an approved new drug, certified antibiotic, or licensed biologic that was marketed as a dietary supplement or food before approval, certification, or license (unless the Secretary of Health and Human Services waives this provision).

If a product or ingredient was already marketed as a dietary supplement prior to 1994, it was "grandfathered" and did not require any notification of the FDA. A new ingredient introduced after the passage of DSHEA, however, must be registered with the FDA as a "new dietary ingredient" (NDI). If a manufacturer wishes to market an NDI, it must notify the FDA with the appropriate safety documentation at least 75 days before marketing it. Appropriate documentation includes information about the chemical identity of the ingredient and justification that the new ingredient "will reasonably be expected to be safe" (DSHEA, 108 Stat 4325 [1994]). The FDA will then respond acknowledging that the file was received and may pose additional questions about the ingredient. The FDA does not "approve" an NDI. By only acknowledging receipt of the premarket filing for an NDI, the FDA reserves the right to have the ingredient removed from the market at its discretion at a later date should it feel it is unsafe. All other nonactive ingredients and excipients used in the manufacture of dietary supplements must be FDA-approved food additives or generally recognized as safe (GRAS).

Safety

Good Manufacturing Practices.   The manufacturing of dietary supplements is regulated by the FDA with the establishment of GMPs similar to those established for foods. GMPs put controls in place over how dietary supplements are manufactured to ensure they are produced in a consistent manner and meet quality standards for identity, purity, concentration, potency, and composition.

The GMPs apply to all domestic and foreign companies that manufacture, package, label, or hold dietary supplements, including those involved with the activities of testing, quality control, packaging and labeling, and distributing them in the United States (21 CFR Part 111). The requirements include provisions related to:

- the design and construction of physical plants that facilitate maintenance and compliance;
- hiring of qualified personnel;
- cleaning and maintenance of manufacturing equipment and facilities;
- proper manufacturing operations;
- quality control procedures and personnel;
- testing the final product and incoming and in-process raw materials;
- handling consumer complaints; and
- maintaining records.

Under DSHEA, the responsibility of ensuring the safety of a dietary supplement falls on the manufacturer. GMPs do not ensure whether a dietary supplement is good for you or not or whether the substance itself is even safe to consume. A dietary supplement is only considered unsafe or "adulterated" if it or one of its ingredients presents "a significant or unreasonable risk of illness or injury" when used as directed on the label or under normal conditions of use when there are no directions. As mentioned with the requirements of premarket notification of NDIs, the FDA does not formally approve dietary supplements before they can be marketed, but under DSHEA, the FDA has the authority to remove any product from the market should it be deemed unsafe. In addition, the manufacturer, bottler, or distributor whose name appears on the label of a dietary supplement marketed in the United States is required to submit to FDA all serious adverse event reports associated with the use of the dietary supplement in the United States (FDA n.d.).

Supplement Labels

FDA regulations require that a descriptive name of the product stating that it is a "dietary supplement" be present on the label. Further, dietary supplement labels must list the ingredient names and amounts in a standardized "supplement facts" panel. The amounts per serving must be listed as a percentage of the Daily Value for each ingredient. Active ingredients that do not have an established Daily Value should also be listed in the supplement facts panel. DSHEA allows the listing of a "proprietary blend" by ingredient without disclosing the amounts of each individual ingredient in the blend. This protects companies using proprietary formulations from having to disclose their formula.

Products are required to meet label claims, which is to say they must contain the levels of active ingredients listed in the supplement facts panel for the duration of the products' shelf life (i.e., up to the date of expiration). Products may be labeled "high potency" if they contain at least 100 percent of the Reference Daily Intake (RDI) for that nutrient. Ingredients that are naturally occurring are allowed to be within 80 percent of the label claim without being considered misbranded. All dietary supplements marketed in the United States must also contain the address and contact information of the manufacturer, packer, or distributor.

Health Benefit Claims

Dietary supplements should not claim or imply that it may be used to treat, mitigate, or cure any disease or illness not directly caused by a nutrient deficiency; more on that later. Statements can be made, however, that describe the role of a nutrient or dietary ingredient intended to affect a structure or function in the body or that characterize the documented mechanism by which a nutrient or dietary ingredient acts to maintain such structure or function, provided that such statements are not disease claims. These are called structure function claims such as those used historically for food and drugs. An example of a structure claim would be, "calcium is important for strong bones and teeth." An example of a function claim might be, "Dietary fiber helps maintain bowel regularity."

FDA regulation stipulates that claims of any type must have adequate substantiation before they can be used to market a dietary supplement. The FDA has stated that it considers two randomized placebo controlled trials of sufficient power and size to be the standard for substantiating a claim. Even an unstated "implied claim" must not be untruthful or misleading and have adequate substantiation. A company must have this substantiation in place before making any health benefit claim to market a product. The FDA must also be notified that you intend to use the claim within 30 days of first marketing the product. All labels that contain health benefit claims must also carry a "disclaimer" that the FDA has not evaluated the claim. The disclaimer must also state that the dietary supplement product is not intended to "diagnose, treat, cure or prevent any disease."

Disease Claims

Disease claims cannot be made for any dietary supplement. A disease claim is defined as any claim, implied or otherwise, that the product is intended to diagnose, mitigate, treat, cure, or prevent any disease. In fact, within DSHEA a drug is not defined by its chemical composition but by the wording used to describe its function. For example, vitamin C can be either a drug or a dietary supplement depending on what you say it will do; thus the statement "Vitamin C may reduce the incidence or duration of a cold" would qualify the product as a new and unapproved drug. Any new or unapproved drug would be required to be removed from the market immediately pending FDA evaluation, again, regardless of what the substance actually is. On the other hand, the statement, "Vitamin C supports the immune system" qualifies the product as a dietary supplement. The one exception for disease claims are nutrient deficiency disease claims. These describe a benefit related to a nutrient deficiency disease (like vitamin D and rickets, or vitamin C and scurvy), but such claims are allowed only if they also inform the consumer of the prevalence of such a disease in the United States.

The Office of Dietary Supplements

The enactment of DSHEA brought with it the creation of the ODS as part of the NIH. The purpose of the ODS is twofold: to explore the potential role of dietary supplements as a significant part of the efforts of the United States to improve health care and to promote scientific study of the benefits of dietary supplements in maintaining health and preventing chronic diseases and other health-related conditions. Though not directly stated, the ODS serves to balance or temper the FDA's long-standing position against dietary supplements by objectively furthering the science and understanding of the role of dietary supplements in public health.

This was only a brief survey of Federal regulation over dietary supplements. For a more in-depth treatment of the subject, the author suggests Wallace's Dietary Supplement Regulation in the United States (Wallace and MacKay 2013). Free access to the DSHEA, and all amendments, is also available through the FDA's website.

Table 1.3 Chronology of federal statutes and amendments on dietary supplements

Year	Statute (amendment)	Citation
1906	PFDA: Adulteration standard that prohibits any added poisonous or deleterious substance injurious to health in food	59th Cong. Sess. 1. Chp. 3915, p. 768–772; cited as 34 U.S. Stats. 768
1938	FDCA: Authorizes foods to bear claims describing effects on a (normal) structure or function of the body; establishes a category of foods for special dietary uses; authorizes the U.S. FDA to regulate such products, which will be deemed misbranded unless the label bears information concerning vitamins, minerals, or other dietary properties as prescribed by FDA regulations as necessary to fully inform purchasers as to the value of the food for such special dietary uses; grants FDA authority to inspect facilities	Public Law 75-717, 52 Stat. 1040
1938	Wheeler–Lea Act: Amends the FTC Act to grant FTC advertising oversight of FDA-regulated products (except prescription drugs)	Public Law 75-447, 52 Stat. 111
1958	Food Additives Amendment: Establishes a premarket approval system for food additives through FDA petition process; defines a food additive as any substance added to food (directly or indirectly), unless the substance is GRAS for its intended use	Public Law 85-929, 72 Stat. 1784

1976	Proxmire Amendment: Prohibits FDA from classifying vitamin and mineral supplements as drugs based solely on their combinations or potency	Public Law 94-278
1990	Nutrition Labeling and Education Act (NLEA): Requires all food labels to contain specific information on the nutritional content (mandates the Nutrition Facts label) and authorizes FDA to consider and permit by regulation claims describing the relationship of specific nutrients to reduced risk of disease (i.e., health claims)	Public Law 101-535
1992	Dietary Supplement Act: Prohibits the implementation of NLEA with respect to dietary supplements except for the approved health claim provision, creating a moratorium to provide Congress and FDA time to draft DSHEA	Public Law 102-6571
1994	DSHEA: Defines the term dietary supplement; exempts dietary ingredients from the food additive provisions in the FDCA; establishes a new safety standard for dietary supplements; and authorizes FDA to impose requirements for GMPs	Public Law 103-417, 108 Stat. 4332
1996	Food Quality Protection Act: Amends the Federal Insecticide, Fungicide, and Rodenticide Act and the FDCA to require complete reassessment of all pesticide tolerances; mandates a single, scientifically based standard for all pesticide tolerances in all foods (including dietary supplements)	Public Law 104-170
1997	Food and Drug Administration Modernization Act (FDAMA): Permits the use of health claims and nutrient content claims based on authoritative statements by a scientific body of the U.S. government (e.g., NIH) provided that premarket notification is sent to FDA	Public Law 105-115
2002	Public Health Security and Bioterrorism Preparedness and Response Act: Requires FDA registration of all food manufacturers and notification in advance of importation of food, including dietary supplements and raw materials	Public Law 107-188
2004	Anabolic Steroid Control Act: Prohibits steroid precursors to be sold in dietary supplements	Public Law 108-358
2004	Food Allergen Labeling and Consumer Protection Act: Requires disclosure on food and dietary supplement labels of 8 major allergens	Public Law 108-132, 118 Stat. 905
2006	Dietary Supplement and Nonprescription Drug Consumer Protection Act: Requires manufacturers and distributors to maintain records of all adverse event reports and to communicate all serious adverse event report data to FDA	Public Law 109-462

(Continued)

Table 1.3 Chronology of federal statutes and amendments on dietary supplements   (Continued)

Year	Statute (amendment)	Citation
2007	Food and Drug Administration Amendments Act: Prohibits the introduction into interstate commerce of any food which contains an added drug	Public Law 110-185
2011	Food Safety Modernization Act (FSMA): Provides FDA with authority to issue a mandatory recall of any food product (except infant formula, which is already subject to FDA mandatory recall authority), including dietary supplements. Other provisions also apply.	Public Law 111-353, 124 Stat. 3885

Source: Adapted from Wallace and MacKay (2013). Dietary supplement regulation in the United States. Used with permission.

References

Adams, S.H. 1911. *The Great American Fraud: Articles on the Nostrum Evil and Quacks, in Two Series.* New York: Collier & Son.

FDA (Food and Drug Administration). n.d. *Dietary Supplements.* www.fda.gov/Food/DietarySupplements/default.htm (accessed March 2015).

Federal Food, Drug, and Cosmetic Act of 1938. 52 Stat 1040, 21 USC §301 et seq.

Fee, E. 2010. "Samuel Hopkins Adams (1871–1958): Journalist and Muckraker." *American Journal of Public Health* 100, no. 8, pp. 1390–91. doi:10.2105/ajph.2009.186452

FDA. 2009. "Data Standards Manual (Monographs): Dosage Form." *FDA.gov.* www.fda.gov/Drugs/DevelopmentApprovalProcess/FormsSubmissionRequirements/ElectronicSubmissions/DataStandardsManualmonographs/ucm071666.htm (accessed August 15, 2015).

Gil-Chávez, G.J., J.A. Villa, J. Fernando Ayala-Zavala, J. Basilio Heredia, D. Sepulveda, E.M. Yahia, and G.A. González-Aguilar. 2013. "Technologies for Extraction and Production of Bioactive Compounds to Be Used as Nutraceuticals and Food Ingredients: An Overview." *Comprehensive Reviews in Food Science and Food Safety* 12, no. 1, pp. 5–23. doi:10.1111/1541-4337.12005

Hutt, P.B. 2005. "FDA Statutory Authority to Regulate the Safety of Dietary Supplements." *American Journal of Law & Medicine* 31, no. 2–3, pp. 155–74. doi:10.1177/009885880503100202

Laird, S.A., A.R. Pierce, and S.F. Schmitt. 2005. "Sustainable Raw Materials in the Botanicals Industry: Constraints and Opportunities." *Acta Horticulturae* 676, pp. 111–17. doi:10.17660/actahortic.2005.676.13

Muth, M.K., D.W. Anderson, J.L. Domanico, J.B. Smith, and B. Wendling. 1999. *Economic Characterization of the Dietary Supplement Industry.* Final, Research Triangle Park, NC: Research Triangle Institute.

Pasupuleti, V.K., and S. Braun. 2010. "State of the Art Manufacturing of Protein Hydrolysates." In *Protein Hydrolysates in Biotechnology*, eds. V.K. Pasupuleti and A.L. Demain, 11–32. New York: Springer Science+Business Media.

Porter, D.V., and R.O. Earl. 1990. "Current Food Labeling." In *Nutrition Labeling: Issues and Directions for the 1990s*, eds. R.O. Earl and D.V. Porter, 51–73. Washington, DC: National Academies Press.

Pure Food and Drug Act of 1906. 34 Stat 768.

Scarbrough, B. 2004. "Dietary Supplements: A Review of United States Regulation with Emphasis on the Dietary Supplement Health and Education Act of 1994 and Subsequent Activity." *Digital Access to Scholarship at Harvard*, Third Year Paper. http://nrs.harvard.edu/urn-3:HUL.InstRepos:8852160 (accessed March 2015).

Simone-Finstrom, M.D., and M. Spivak. 2012. "Increased Resin Collection After Parasite Challenge: A Case of Self-Medication in Honey Bees?" *PLoS One* 7, no. 3: e34601. doi:10.1371/journal.pone.0034601

Wallace, T.C., and D. MacKay. 2013. "Dietary Supplement Regulation in the United States." In *SpringerBriefs in Food, Health, and Nutrition*, eds. T.C. MacKay, D. Al-Mondhiry, R. Nguyen, H. Griffiths, and J.C. Wallace, 1–38. Cham: Springer International Publishing.

Young, J.H. 1972. *The Toadstool Millionaires: A Social History of Patent Medicines in America Before Federal Regulation.* Princeton, NJ: Princeton University Press.

CHAPTER 2

Survey of the 20 Most Common Dietary Supplements— Vitamins and Minerals

Overview

This chapter reviews 5 of the 20 most popular supplements. This chapter focuses on vitamin and mineral products formulated into multivitamin mineral blends as well as other widely applicable individual nutrients such as vitamin D, Calcium, vitamin C, and the B vitamins. Their function in the body is discussed as well as the primary motivations or health benefits driving their use. Safety is also reviewed.

Introduction

Having explored dietary supplements by formal definitions, manufacturing methods, and federal regulations, we now turn our attention to the 20 most popular dietary supplements. By popular we mean those that are purchased and consumed by the largest numbers of people in the United States. The list was compiled by the Council for Responsible Nutrition,[1]

---

[1] All market data comes from the 2014 CRN Consumer Survey on Dietary Supplements, conducted August 25–29, 2014, by Ipsos Public Affairs, and funded by CRN. The survey was conducted online and included a national sample of 2,010 adults aged 18 and older from Ipsos' U.S. online panel. The survey has been conducted annually since 2000. Weighting was employed to balance demographics and ensure that the sample's composition reflects that of the U.S. adult population according to Census data and to provide results intended to approximate the sample universe. For more information, visit: www.crnusa.org/CRNconsumersurvey/2014
Source: Council for Responsible Nutrition.

and it might surprise you. It is likely you are already familiar with some and not so much with others. We discuss what each supplement is, where it comes form, how it functions in the body, and the most common reasons that people take it for.

We have attempted to provide evidence produced by clinical trials in support of benefit claims wherever possible. You will find, however, as is often the case in academia, that the question of efficacy is not always black and white. Nor is our treatment of each ingredient comprehensive. The scope of such an endeavor is far beyond the scope of this book. Nevertheless, it was our intention to present the information in as clear and objective a manner as possible.

The 20 most popular supplements are divided into four categories: vitamins and minerals, specialty supplements, herbs and botanicals, and sports nutrition and weight management. Within these four categories are found a wide variety of compounds ranging from simple macro and micronutrients to natural drug-like compounds extracted from herbs called nutraceuticals. Vitamins and minerals are by far the most popular within our list with 97 percent of all consumers who use dietary supplements using vitamins and minerals. Specialty supplements are next in rank of popularity with 43 percent of supplement consumers using them. Herbs and botanicals follow next with 26 percent of consumers taking some form of herbal product. Finally, sports and weight management (i.e., loss) products with 19 percent of all supplement users taking them.

Multivitamin and Mineral Supplements

Background

Over half of the U.S. population takes some form of dietary supplement, the most common supplements being multivitamin and mineral (MVM) products (Gahche et al. 2011). The first product of this kind was produced and marketed in the 1930s by the Nutrilite Company (NIH, State-of-the-Science Panel 2007; Wallace 2013). At that time, a MVM supplement was simply vegetable and fruit juice concentrates dried and compressed into a tablet. Today, the majority of vitamins and minerals are produced chemically (i.e., synthetically) or by fermentation (Muth 1999). This is of course by necessity as the task of extracting vitamins and minerals from food sources would be impossible due to the large volumes consumed each year. For example, global production of vitamin C is ~110,000 metric tons annually (Board 2012). Considering that an average sized orange has ~60 mg vitamin C, if you were to try to extract all the vitamin C we consume each year, it would require over 1 trillion oranges; so chemical synthesis is an absolute necessity to meet the demand.

MVMs are very popular dietary supplements and, according to estimates, more than one-third of all Americans take them in some form (NIH, State-of-the-Science Panel 2007). MVMs account for almost one-sixth of all purchases of dietary supplements and 40 percent of all sales of vitamin and mineral supplements. Sales of all dietary supplements in the United States totaled an estimated $36.7 billion in 2014. This amount included $14.3 billion for all vitamin- and mineral-containing supplements, of which $5.7 billion was for MVMs (NIH, Office of Dietary Supplements 2015).

An MVM product may have all essential vitamins and minerals or only a selection. They may have 100 percent of the Daily Value (DV) for each nutrient, or much more, or much less. For a list of essential vitamins and minerals and their DV, see Table 2.1. The possible combinations for an MVM are nearly limitless. You will also see products combining vitamins, minerals, and botanicals or herbal extracts.

A recent trend is to market specific blends of vitamins and minerals to certain consumer groups. For example, a "One a Day Multi for Women" would be a simple multivitamin mineral blend but with additional calcium and vitamin D. Claims about bone mass and its importance for women's health would be based on the extra calcium and vitamin D. Likewise, a common strategy for a men's product is a similar multivitamin blend but with an herbal extract from a plant called Saw Palmetto. Saw Palmetto is believed to support prostate health, and as men are the only gender that has a prostate, it makes an easy story to target the product towards men.

Rationale for Supplementation

The primary reason people take MVMs is as insurance against possible dietary deficiencies. The concern is not unwarranted. According to the

Table 2.1 *Vitamin and mineral DV based on a caloric intake of 2,000 calories, for adults and children four or more years of age and upper tolerable intake level (UL)*

Vitamin or mineral	Function	DV 100%	UL for healthy adults
Vitamin A	Vision, immunity, skin, body growth	5,000 International Units (IU)	10,000 IU
Vitamin C	Collagen synthesis, fat metabolism, antioxidant defense, mood	60 mg	2,000 mg
Calcium (Ca)	Bone growth and bone density, cell function	1,000 mg	2,500 mg
Iron (Fe)	A factor in red blood cell formation and function of hemoglobin	18 mg	45 mg
Vitamin D	Bone growth and density, immunity, blood sugar, blood pressure (BP)	400 IU	333.3 IU
Vitamin E	Antioxidant defense, immunity	30 IU	111 IU
Vitamin K	Proper blood clotting, bone growth and bone density	80 μg	Not Determinable (ND)
Vitamin B1 (thiamine)	Energy production from food	1.5 mg	ND
Vitamin B2 (riboflavin)	Energy production from food, metabolism of protein, carbohydrates, and fat, antioxidant defense	1.7 mg	ND
Vitamin B3 (niacin)	Energy production from food, cell signaling	20 mg	35 mg
Vitamin B6	Nervous system function, red blood cell production and function, hormone regulation	2 mg	100 mg
Folate (folic acid)	DNA production, DNA and RNA function, amino acid metabolism, mood	400 μg	1,000 μg
Vitamin B12	Hemoglobin production, DNA and RNA function, amino acid metabolism, mood	6 μg	ND
Biotin	Metabolism of certain amino acids, cholesterol, and fatty acids, DNA and cell replication	300 μg	ND

Nutrient	Function		
Pantothenic acid	Energy production from food, fat, cholesterol, hormone, and neurotransmitter production, DNA and cell replication, gene expression, nerve function	10 mg	ND
Phosphorus (P)	Plays a central role in energy and cell metabolism, acid base balance	1,000 mg	4,000 mg
Iodine (I)	Thyroid activity and metabolic rate	150 µg	1,100 µg
Magnesium (Mg)	Over 300 essential metabolic reactions and cell functions. Bone density	400 mg	350 mg*
Zinc (Zn)	Cellular metabolism, gene expression, normal growth and development, immunity, neurological function, and reproduction	15 mg	40 mg
Selenium (Se)	Essential component of the enzyme glutathione peroxidase, protects cellular tissues and membranes against oxidative damage	70 µg	400 µg
Copper (Cu)	Essential component of oxidation–reduction enzyme systems, iron metabolism, hemoglobin synthesis, and red blood cell production and maintenance, skin pigmentation, formation of bone and connective tissue, and integrity of the myelin sheath of nerve fibers	2 mg	10 mg
Manganese (Mn)	Cofactor or component of several key enzyme systems, bone formation, regeneration of red blood cells, carbohydrate metabolism, and the reproductive cycle	2 mg	11 mg
Chromium (Cr)	Insulin action, cholesterol and amino acid metabolism	120 µg	ND
Molybdenum (Mo)	Cofactor in the active site of four enzymes: sulfite oxidase, xanthine oxidase, aldehyde oxidase, and mitochondrial amidoxime reducing component	75 µg	2,000 µg
Chloride (Cl)	Regulation of osmotic pressure and acid-base balance, transport of oxygen and carbon dioxide in the blood, maintenance of gastric acidity level (pH)	3,400 mg	3,600 mg
Sodium (Na)	Electrolyte, nerve function, regulation of osmotic pressure and the maintenance of acid–base balance, muscle excitability, absorption of carbohydrate	2,400 mg	2,300 mg
Potassium (K)	Regulation of intracellular osmotic pressure and acid–base balance, muscle excitability, glycogen and protein synthesis, glycolysis.	3,500 mg	ND

*From dietary supplements only.

Office of Disease Prevention and Health Promotion, many of us are not eating adequate amounts of vitamin A, vitamin D, vitamin E, folate, vitamin C, calcium, and magnesium. Iron is underconsumed by adolescent and premenopausal females, including women who are pregnant, and potassium and fiber are underconsumed relative to the suggested adequate intake. It's important to keep in mind that caloric content of a diet does not reflect its nutritional adequacy.

It is clear that taking an MVM supplement can ensure that we are getting adequate amounts of vitamins and minerals while consuming a less than adequate diet. What isn't clear is the impact that MVM supplementation has on disease prevention. The available research on the long term impact of MVM use and disease is insufficient to make a definitive statement one way or the other. There is, for example, some evidence that bone mineral density may be beneficially affected long term in menopausal women. Protection from illness and various cancers, however, has yet to be clearly demonstrated. Perhaps the best evidence to date comes from a recent study conducted by the Office of Dietary Supplements that found an association between MVM use (>3 years) and reduced cardiovascular disease (CVD) mortality risk for women after controlling for various confounding factors (Bailey 2015). Interestingly, the same benefit was not seen in men.

One problem faced by academics when trying to elucidate the role of chronic vitamin and mineral supplementation is the wide variety of products and formulas that fall into that category. This is evident even in published research. For example, the Agency for Healthcare Research and Quality, in a review of the evidence for the role of MVM supplements in chronic disease prevention, defined MVMs as "any supplement containing three or more vitamins and minerals but no herbs, hormones, or drugs, with each component at a dose less than the tolerable upper level determined by the Food and Nutrition Board ..." (Huang 2006; NIH, Office of Dietary Supplements 2015). Another study defined MVMs more ambiguously as "stress-tab-type," "therapeutic or theragran type," and "one-a-day" type (Lawson 2007). Studying the disease-preventing potential from long term use of products containing multiple vitamins and minerals is not likely to produce reliable data in the near future. The variables are just too numerous.

Safety

Taking an MVM that provides nutrients at or below recommended intakes should pose no safety risk to healthy people. Safety becomes a concern, however, when one or more ingredients meet or exceed the established ULs for vitamins and minerals. The Food and Nutrition board of the Institutes of Medicine has published ULs for most essential vitamins and minerals (see Table 2.1). The greatest risk of overdose comes from the fat-soluble vitamins. Water-soluble vitamins are excreted relatively easily when intake exceeds the body's need and for this reason most water-soluble vitamins do not have an established UL. Fat soluble vitamins, however, are stored in the liver and fatty tissues in the body and can rise to toxic levels if intake exceeds the body's ability to use them; a classic example is developing vitamin A toxicity from eating too much liver (i.e., hypervitaminosis) (Shearman 1978). The greatest risk of adverse events from taking MVM products comes from those products that contain additional non-nutrient ingredients such as herbal extracts, which can have drug like properties.

Drug interaction is also an important concern. Unlike many herbal extracts, most vitamins and minerals do not pose significant risk of interaction with prescription medications; one notable exception being vitamin K and anticoagulant drugs such as Coumadin.

Vitamin D

Background

Vitamin D is a fat-soluble hormone-like vitamin that is naturally present in a limited number of foods (see Table 2.2). Because of its relative scarcity even in a well-balanced diet, it is added to some foods such as milk and breakfast cereals. Foods to which vitamins or minerals have been added are referred to as fortified foods. It is also available as a dietary supplement. Vitamin D in dietary supplements is provided in one of two forms, vitamin D2 (ergocalciferol) or vitamin D3 (cholecalciferol). The majority of the daily requirement for vitamin D is met through endogenous production. When ultraviolet rays from sunlight strike the skin, Vitamin D synthesis is triggered.

Table 2.2 Food sources of vitamin D

Food	IU	DV (%)
Swordfish, cooked, 3 ounces	566	142
Salmon (sockeye), cooked, 3 ounces	447	112
Tuna fish, canned in water, drained, 3 ounces	154	39
Orange juice fortified with vitamin D, 1 cup (amount of added vitamin D varies by brand)	137	34
Milk, nonfat, reduced fat, and whole, vitamin D-fortified, 1 cup	115–124	29–31
Yogurt, fortified with 20% of the DV for vitamin D, 6 ounces (more heavily fortified yogurts provide more of the DV)	80	20
Margarine, fortified, 1 tablespoon	60	15
Sardines, canned in oil, drained, 2 sardines	46	12
Liver, beef, cooked, 3 ounces	42	11
Egg, 1 large (vitamin D is found in yolk)	41	10
Ready-to-eat cereal, fortified with 10% of the DV for vitamin D, 0.75–1 cup (more heavily fortified cereals might provide more of the DV)	40	10
Cheese, Swiss, 1 ounce	6	2

Source: U.S. Department of Agriculture, Agricultural Research Service (2011). USDA National Nutrient Database for Standard Reference, Release 24.

Vitamin D increases calcium absorption from the intestine and maintains adequate serum calcium and phosphate concentrations to enable normal mineralization of bone and to prevent hypocalcemic tetany. It is also needed for bone growth and bone remodeling by osteoblasts and osteoclasts. Without sufficient vitamin D, bones become demineralized causing them to become thin, brittle, or misshapen. Together with calcium, vitamin D also helps protect against the loss of bone mineral density as we age.

Vitamin D2 or vitamin D3 obtained from sun exposure, food or a fortified food, or a supplement is biologically inert and must undergo hydroxylation twice in the body for activation. The first occurs in the liver converting vitamin D to the prehormone 25-hydroxyvitamin D

(25(OH)D). This inactive form is the main metabolite circulating in the blood and is used for the classification of vitamin D status (Bouillon et al. 2008; Holick 2007). Vitamin D is further hydroxylated to its most active form, the calcium regulating secosteroid hormone 1,25-dihydroxy-vitamin D (1,25(OH)2D) by the enzyme, 1-α-hydroxylase, also known as calcitriol, predominantly in the kidneys. 1-α-hydroxylase is also found to be active in extrarenal tissues throughout the body (Organization 2012) giving rise to the assumption that vitamin D plays a widespread role in the overall health, including that of tissues such as those of the heart and the blood vessels (Kienreich et al. 2013).

Calcitriol, produced in the kidneys or extrarenally in other target tissues (Forman et al. 2013), is the ligand of the vitamin D receptor (VDR), whose widespread distribution across many tissues explains the myriad of physiological actions of vitamin D. By interacting with the VDR, a transcription factor, calcitriol regulates directly and indirectly the expression of over 200 genes (Ramagopalan 2010).

Rationale for Supplementation

The DV for vitamin D is currently set at 400 IU for adults and children age four and older. Probably the most well-known disease attributed to vitamin D deficiency is rickets. Rickets is characterized by bone pain or tenderness, increased incidence of bone fractures, impaired growth in children, muscle cramps and pronounced muscle weakness, dental deformities, skeletal deformities such as an odd-shaped skull, bowlegs, deformed ribcage, pelvic deformities, and spine deformities (including scoliosis or kyphosis). Signs of improvement in an individual with rickets can be seen in as little as one week with generous vitamin D and mineral supplementation.

Although rickets is extremely rare in developed countries, vitamin D *insufficiency* is highly prevalent; this is reflected in the fact that more than half of the population worldwide has levels below 30 ng/mL (Mithal et al. 2009; Van Schoor and Lips 2011). Different factors, such as increased age, being female, darker skin pigmentation, reduced sun exposure, as well as seasonal variation and distance from the equator, are all risk factors for vitamin D insufficiency. The increasing prevalence of low levels of vitamin D is also explainable by changes in lifestyle and, to some extent, by air pollution.

Cardiovascular (CV) risk factors, such as arterial hypertension, obesity, dyslipidemia, or diabetes mellitus, as well as myocardial infarction, coronary artery disease, or stroke, are the most prevalent conditions and account for the major causes of death worldwide, especially in Western countries (Organization 2012). The prospective Intermountain Heart Collaborative Study with more than 40,000 participants revealed that vitamin D insufficiency was associated with highly significant increases in the prevalence of type 2 diabetes mellitus, hypertension, hyperlipid-emia, and peripheral vascular disease, coronary artery disease, myocardial infarction, heart failure, and stroke, as well as with incident death (all-cause mortality was used as primary survival measure) (Anderson et al. 2010).

Essential hypertension is related to several disturbances in the sys-temic and cellular calcium metabolism. Vitamin D status may be a risk factor for hypertension. A large meta-analysis assessing the association of baseline vitamin D status with the risk of hypertension was performed by Kunutsor, Apekey, and Steur (2013). They included 11 prospective studies published between 2005 and 2012, which comprised a total of 283,537 participants and 55,816 cases of hypertension with a mean follow-up of 9 years (Kunutsor, Apekey, and Steur 2013). The authors reported on a significant inverse association of baseline circulating serum vitamin D levels with the risk of incident hypertension. When evaluating dose–response in five studies that reported risk ratios (RRs) for vitamin D exposure, the authors found that the risk for hypertension was lowered by 12 percent per 10 ng/mL increment of 25(OH)D (Kunutsor, Apekey, and Steur 2013). This was the largest meta-analysis performed giving strong evidence for a relationship between vitamin D and BP.

Several randomized controlled trials have been performed to evaluate the effect of vitamin D on BP levels in various cohorts with varying results (Forman et al. 2013; Larsen et al. 2012; Wood et al. 2012). Larsen performed a randomized controlled trial in 130 hypertensive patients who were given supplements of 3,000 IU of vitamin D or placebo over 20 weeks during winter in Denmark. They found a nonsignificant reduction of BP in the results of 24-hour ambulatory BP monitoring.

Interestingly, when only vitamin D-insufficient patients were analyzed, with vitamin D levels below 32 ng/mL, systolic and diastolic BP levels in 24-hour ambulatory BP monitoring were significantly lowered in the therapy group compared to the placebo group (Larsen et al. 2012). This effect in hypertensive and vitamin D-deficient patients has also been seen in a study by Forman et al., who performed a randomized controlled trial in black Americans, who are known to be at a very high risk of both vitamin D deficiency and hypertension (Forman et al. 2013). They included 283 participants who were given 1,000, 2,000, or 4,000 IU of vitamin D or placebo over three months. They were able to show that supplementation of vitamin D led to a reduction of 0.2 mmHg of systolic BP for each increase of 1 ng/mL of vitamin D over three months. These results indicate the effect of vitamin D supplementation on BP, particularly in vitamin D-insufficient or deficient individuals.

Clinical trials have shown positive effects of vitamin D and its analogues on fibrinolysis, blood lipids, thrombogenicity, endothelial regeneration, and smooth muscle cell growth (Dobnig et al. 2008; Ku et al. 2013; Michos and Melamed 2008). Together, this data indicates that vitamin D has beneficial effects that are independent of calcium metabolism.

Several mechanisms might be responsible for the protective effect of vitamin D on atherosclerotic lesions and vascular calcification. First, vascular smooth cells express VDRs. Vitamin D inhibits proliferation of smooth muscle cells (Wu-Wong et al. 2006). Second, a lack of vitamin D results in an increase in the serum parathyroid hormone (PTH) levels. Excess PTH levels may promote CVD by increasing the cardiac contractility and myocardial calcification (Rostand and Drüeke 1999). Third, in vitro studies have shown that vitamin D suppresses the release of the inflammatory cytokines. There is now increasing evidence that inflammation plays an important role in the development of a vascular damage (Sullivan, Sarembock, and Linden 2000). Fourth, vitamin D is a negative endocrine regulator of the renin-angiotensin-aldosterone system. The renin-angiotensin-aldosterone system plays a central role in the regulation of BP, electrolytes, and blood volume. Vitamin D treatment reduces BP, plasma renin activity, and angiotensin II levels (Li et al. 2002). Fifth, vascular smooth muscle cell proliferation and migration, as well as the osteogenic processes may contribute to the vascular calcification, which may lead to a thrombotic event (Gunta, Thadhani, and Mak 2013). Sixth, vitamin D plays a role in insulin sensitivity, which has a role in diabetes and in metabolic syndrome.

Hyperlipidemia, diabetic mellitus, and an increase in blood coagulation factors, blood viscosity, and leukocyte counts are important risk factors for the development of arteriosclerosis. There is now increasing evidence that arteriosclerosis is a low-grade systemic inflammatory disease. An increase in serum C-reactive protein levels is an important indicator of inflammatory reactions and the risk of developing arteriosclerosis (Van Lente 2000). Calcitriol can suppress the secretion of TNF-α and IL-6 in vitro in a dose-dependent manner (Mendall et al. 1997). A recent study identified an inverse association between TNF-α and vitamin D levels in human subjects (Zittermann et al. 2003).

Based on systematic reviews and meta-analyses of the currently available literature, it can be concluded that vitamin D deficiency is an independent CV risk factor that is associated with increased risk of CV events. However, it is largely unclear whether these associations are causal in nature. While it seems plausible that vitamin D deficiency can be considered a surrogate marker for poorer health status, most notably observed in patients with chronic diseases, including CV risk factors and CVD, it remains to be proven whether vitamin D itself can directly impact CV outcomes (Kienreich et al. 2013; McGreevy and Williams 2011). What continues to be needed are randomized controlled trials using sufficiently high doses of vitamin D to clearly see the effect on various health outcomes. However, the existing body of evidence from in vitro, ecological, case-control, retrospective, and prospective observational and interventional studies is substantial and suggests a pivotal role of vitamin D for a variety of physiological functions and health outcomes, particularly CV health.

Safety

A daily intake of 600 IUs per day or a serum level of ≥50 nmol/L (≥20 ng/mL) vitamin D is considered adequate to meet the nutritional needs of 97.5 percent of people. The UL for vitamin D has been set at 4,000 IU by the Institute of Medicine, Food and Nutrition Board. Similarly a serum level of >125 nmol/L (>50 ng/mL) vitamin D is an upper threshold and has been associated with adverse effects. Vitamin D toxicity manifests itself with symptoms such as anorexia, weight loss, polyuria, and heart arrhythmias. Theoretically, too much vitamin D may lead to excess calcium in the blood (hypercalcemia), which may increase arterial calcification and subsequent damage to the heart, blood vessels, and kidney.

Few studies have been conducted to evaluate the safety of high dose vitamin D supplementation. Most reports suggest that the toxicity threshold is far above 4,000 IUs/day. 10,000 to 40,000 IUs/day is where most data points to a toxicity threshold. Nevertheless, the Food and Nutrition Board advises that recent data points to the possibility of adverse events even at lower intakes below the UL in the long term. The Food and Nutrition Board committee pointed to research which found that vitamin D intakes of 5,000 IU/day achieved serum vitamin D levels between 100 to 150 nmol/L (40 to 60 ng/mL), but no greater. Applying an uncertainty factor of 20 percent to this intake value gave an upper limit of 4,000 IU, which the Food and Nutrition Board applied to individuals aged nine and older.

Calcium

Background

Calcium is the most abundant mineral found in the body. The largest store of calcium in the body, ~99 percent, is incorporated into the skeleton. This concentration is active on a daily basis, with about 0.5 g of calcium moving out of and being deposited back into the bones each day. Skeletal calcium has two important functions: it is the scaffolding for a rigid framework that helps protect internal organs and facilitates movement, and it provides a pool of available calcium for times when intestinal absorption and renal conservation are not sufficient to fulfill the body's need for calcium. The physiological functions of calcium are fundamental to survival; consequently, all living things have evolved strong mechanisms specifically to maintain constant intracellular and extracellular calcium concentrations. These mechanisms are controlled by interactions between the

PTH, calcitonin, and calcitriol (1,25-dihydroxycholecalciferol). Calcium also acts as a second messenger, allowing cells to respond to stimuli such as hormones and neurotransmitters. Calcium is also an important molecule in the activation of hydrolytic enzymes, most notably those that hydrolyze polysaccharides, phospholipids, and proteins.

Calcium is a divalent cation. Within the cell, most calcium is stored in organelles such as the nucleus, vesicles, and the endoplasmic reticulum. The electrochemical gradient of calcium across the cell membrane is about 10,000 fold. Any release of calcium from organelles or transport across the cell membrane into the cytosol triggers a large increase in cytosolic calcium concentration. These changes act as intracellular messengers that help regulate various cellular functions, including skeletal and heart muscle contraction, hormonal secretion, glycogen metabolism, and cell division (Nathanson 1994; Rasmussen 1986).

Extracellular calcium also has important functions in the body. Homeostasis of this calcium pool is tightly regulated by a system involving the parathyroid glands and calcium-transporting cells in the intestine, skeleton, and kidney (Stewart and Broadus 1987). This system helps maintain a steady supply of calcium for the vital intracellular functions. Physiological functions of extracellular calcium include maintenance of intracellular adhesion and integrity of the plasma membrane, as well as support for blood clotting.

Table 2.3 contains a list of food sources of dietary calcium. Whenever possible, nutrient deficiencies are best met with a nutrient-rich diet. Most people however find it difficult to meet all of their nutritional needs through diet alone, so they turn to dietary supplements. The most common forms of calcium found in dietary supplements are calcium lactate, citrate, gluconate, and carbonate. The first three forms of calcium have better absorption profiles than the carbonate form, and this is particularly important in the elderly population and those suffering from hypochlorhydria. Calcium carbonate is the least expensive form, but its value is limited due to its poor bioavailability. Various foods taken with calcium supplements can also have an effect on the mineral's absorption. Fiber-rich foods including bran, whole-grain cereals, and breads are rich in phytates, which can impede calcium absorption. Conversely, lactose rich foods, namely dairy products, can improve the absorption of calcium.

Table 2.3 Food sources of calcium

Food	Calcium (mg) per measure	DV (%)
Orange juice, frozen concentrate, unsweetened, undiluted with added Ca (1 cup)	1,514	151
Seeds, sesame seeds, whole, dried (1 cup)	1,404	140
Seeds, *sisymbrium* sp. seeds, whole, dried (1 cup)	1,208	121
Whey, acid, dried (1 cup)	1,171	117
Milk, dry, whole, without added vitamin D (1 cup)	1,167	117
Whey, sweet, dried (1 cup)	1,154	115
Cheese, parmesan, dry grated, reduced fat (1 cup)	1,109	111
Cheese, mozzarella, nonfat (1 cup)	1,086	109
Cheese, pasteurized process, Swiss (1 cup)	1,081	108
Cheese, Swiss (1 cup diced)	1,044	104
USDA Commodity, cheese, cheddar, reduced fat (1 cup shredded)	1,023	102
General Mills Total Raisin Bran (1 cup)	1,000	100
General Mills, Whole Grain Total (3/4 cup)	1,000	100
Cheese, provolone, reduced fat (1 cup diced)	998	99
Cheese, provolone (1 cup diced)	998	99
Cheese, Monterey (1 cup diced)	985	98
Cheese, mozzarella, low sodium (1 cup diced)	965	96
Cheese, pasteurized processed, American, low fat (1 cup diced)	958	96
Cheese, pasteurized processed, Swiss, low fat (1 cup diced)	958	96
Cheese, Muenster (1 cup diced)	946	95
Cheese, mozzarella, low moisture, part-skim (1 cup diced)	945	95
Cheese, Monterey, low fat (1 cup diced)	931	93
Cheese, low-sodium, cheddar or Colby (1 cup diced)	928	93
Cheese, Colby (1 cup diced)	904	90
Restaurant, Italian, lasagna with meet (1 serving)	900	90

Source: U.S. Department of Agriculture, Agricultural Research Service (2011). USDA National Nutrient Database for Standard Reference, Release 27.

Taking calcium supplements in divided doses 60 to 90 minutes after a meal may also improve the overall absorption.

Rationale for Supplementation

Dietary Calcium intake is generally inadequate in the United States, most notably in the populations with the greatest needs. The U.S. FDA Total Diet Study estimated the intakes of 11 nutritional elements by specific age–sex groups in the United States (Pennington and Schoen 1996). Results showed that there is a need for concern about dietary intakes of calcium, among other minerals, for some age–sex categories. The intake levels were somewhat low for older males, but were only 61 to 78 percent of the Recommended Dietary Allowance (RDA) for two-year-olds and for all of the female subgroups.

Because of these low intake levels, the FDA has classified dietary intake of calcium as a public health problem. The RDA for Calcium ranges from 1,000 to 1,300 mg/day for individuals 4 years of age and older. During the preteen and teenage years (9 to 18 years), recommended levels are increased to 1,300 mg/day for males and females, to provide adequate calcium to support the formation of strong bones. The levels are again increased during the older years (>70 years for males and 51 years plus for females) to help maintain bone mass and to help compensate for decreased intake levels (Institute of Medicine (U.S.) Standing Committee on the Scientific Evaluation of Dietary Reference Intakes 1997).

Calcium supplementation is most commonly recommended for the maintenance of bone health during the formative years, for the prevention of osteoporosis, and for the preservation of bone mineral density with age (Foundation 2010; Warensjo et al. 2011). Bone growth is at its peak during the teenage years, and bone density remains relatively constant throughout the adult years. In women, after age 40, bone loss occurs at a rate of 0.5 to 1 percent per year typically. The same decline is detected in men, but usually occurs several decades later than in women. When dietary calcium intake levels are low, as is the case for many Americans, bone loss is more pronounced (Bryant, Cadogan, and Weaver 1999). Dietary intakes of calcium, and the serum calcium levels related to them, are tightly associated with levels of calcium in the bone. When serum calcium levels decline, PTH levels increase, stimulating osteoclasts to break down bone to pull calcium from the bones into the blood. In contrast, calcium supplementation can inhibit increases in PTH, and reduce bone loss in these cases. In premenopausal women (18 to 50 years old), 1,000 mg supplemental calcium per day may reduce bone loss (Welten et al. 1995). Immediately postmenopause, calcium supplementation may be less beneficial, due to rapid estrogen losses decreasing intestinal calcium absorption. Estrogen treatment may help reduce bone loss during this time, and calcium may have an additive effect in this case (Nieves et al. 1998). Five years post-menopause, calcium supplementation begins to have a significant benefit on bone health again. Supplementation with 1,000 to 1,600 mg of calcium daily during this time period may reduce bone loss from 2 percent annually without calcium supplementation to 0.25 to 1 percent annually (Nordin 2009). It is estimated that daily calcium supplementation for 30 years after menopause might result in a 10 percent improvement in bone mineral density, and a 26 to 70 percent overall reduction in fracture rates, compared with women who do not take calcium supplements (Chiu 1999; Cumming and Nevitt 1997).

Less commonly, calcium is also used to prevent premenstrual syndrome (PMS) and to reduce the risk of colorectal cancer. Calcium carbonate is also commonly used as an antacid. Low calcium intakes may trigger symptoms of PMS, and women consuming around 1,200 mg of calcium per day seem to have ~30 percent lower risk of developing PMS compared to women consuming an average of around 500 mg of calcium daily (Bertone-Johnson et al. 2005). Supplementation around 1,000 mg of calcium daily may significantly reduce several PMS symptoms, including depressed mood, water retention, and pain and has been shown to decrease overall symptom scores by about 18 percent compared with placebo (Alvir and Thys-Jacobs 1991; Penland and Johnson 1993; Thys-Jacobs et al. 1998). Population studies have uncovered an association between high calcium intake via supplementation or the diet and a reduced risk of colorectal cancer or colorectal adenoma recurrence (Carroll et al. 2010; Cooper et al. 2010). There is some research, however, that does not support this association. Finally, calcium has been shown to be effective as an antacid for the treatment of dyspepsia, and the FDA has approved calcium carbonate for this use (Maton and Burton 1999).

Safety

Calcium is safe when supplemented in appropriate dosages, but dosages exceeding the Tolerable Upper Limit (TUL) may increase the risk of significant side effects such as hypercalcemia or milk-alkali syndrome. By age group, the TULs for Calcium are: 0 to 6 months, 1,000 mg; 6 to 12 months, 1,500 mg; 1 to 8 years, 2,500 mg; 9 to 18 years, 3,000 mg; 19 to 50 years, 2,500 mg; 51+ years, 2,000 mg/day (Abrams 2010). Calcium intakes ranging from 1,000 to 2,500 mg daily do not result in hypercalciuria in normal individuals; however, some individuals with hypercalciuria or other similar diseases may exhibit hyperabsorption of calcium and should avoid calcium supplements. Patients with a history of urinary tract stones should consult their physician before supplementing their diet with calcium.

Recently, concern has arisen around the potential negative effects of excessive calcium intakes via dietary supplements and the risk of arterial calcification and CVD in older individuals (Anderson and Klemmer 2013). The concern is that even healthy kidneys have a limited capability to remove excess calcium from the blood, and this capacity declines with age. Excess calcium not removed from the bloodstream may result in soft-tissue calcification, increasing the risk for CVD. While bone health maintenance is an important concern in the aging population, the risk of excess calcium, increasing the risk of CVD, must be considered when recommending calcium supplements to the aging population.

A major drug interaction rating has been identified for calcium and Ceftriaxone (Rocephin) (Bradley et al. 2009). These two compounds should not be taken in combination. Moderate drug interaction ratings exist for calcium with Aluminum Salts, Bisphosphonates, Calcipotriene (Dovonex), Digoxin (Lanoxin), Diltiazem (Cardizem, Dilacor, Tiazac), Levothyroxine (Synthroid, Levothroid, Levoxyl), Lithium, Quinolone and Tetracycline Antibiotics, Sotalol (Betapace), Thiazide Diuretics, and Verapamil (Calan, Covera, Isoptin, Verelan). (Calcium *Professional Monograph*) Individuals should be cautious and consult their health care provider regarding these combinations.

Vitamin C

Background

Vitamin C is a water-soluble vitamin, meaning it is not stored long term in the body. Excess amounts are excreted from the body via the urine. Vitamin C is an essential nutrient, as we lack the enzyme L-gulonolactone oxidase used to synthesize vitamin C from glucose, which means humans need to obtain all of their vitamin C through the diet. Few mammals lack this ability, namely humans, primates, guinea pigs, and fruit bats. Vitamin C is found in many foods, but most commonly in fruits and vegetables (see Table 2.4 for the top 25 sources). It is also available as a dietary supplement. Vitamin C in dietary supplements is most commonly provided as ascorbic acid and may be combined with calcium, magnesium, and potassium mineral ascorbates to offer a buffered form that is easier on sensitive stomachs. Ascorbic acid can be extracted from natural sources, most commonly corn starch, corn sugar, or rice starch, or it may be synthesized in a laboratory from sugars such as glucose.

Vitamin C deficiency, or scurvy, is rare in the industrialized world, but was a common occurrence among sailors, pirates, and others who were at sea for long periods of time without access to fresh fruits and vegetables. Symptoms of scurvy include listlessness, malaise, changes in personality and psychomotor performance, frail hair, bleeding gums and gingivitis, poor wound healing, bone pain and fractures, chest pain, thickened pericardium, thrombosis, and other CV effects (Bender 2003).

When consumed orally, vitamin C is absorbed in the intestines and transported throughout the body via sodium-dependent vitamin C transporters, SVCT1, and SVCT2. SVCT1 is found in the lining of the intestines and is responsible for intestinal uptake and renal reabsorption of vitamin C to support homeostasis. SVCT2 is found in specialized tissues and carries vitamin C to the tissues that use it for enzymatic reactions or require it for antioxidant support (Savini et al. 2008; Tsukaguchi et al. 1999). Excess vitamin C is excreted from the body via the urine most commonly as dehydroascorbate, ketogulonate, ascorbate 2-sulfate,

Table 2.4 Food sources of vitamin C

Food	Vitamin C per serving (mg)	DV (%)
Acerola juice, raw	3,872	6,453
Acerola, (West Indian cherry), raw	1,644	2,740
Rose hips, wild (Northern Plains, Indian)	541	901
Orange juice, frozen concentrate, unsweetened, undiluted, with added calcium	379.4	632
Orange juice, frozen concentrate, unsweetened, undiluted	379.4	632
Guavas, common, raw	376.7	628
Guava sauce, cooked	348.4	581
Peppers, sweet, yellow, raw	341.3	569
Juice Smoothie, Bothouse Farms, Berry Boost	273.7	456
Formulated Bar, Mars Snackfood US, Snickers Marathon Energy Bar, all flavors	269.4	449
Grapefruit Juice, white, frozen concentrate, unsweetened, undiluted	248	413
Peaches, frozen, sliced, sweetened	235.5	393
Peppers, sweet, red, cooked, boiled, drained, without salt	230.8	385
Pokeberry shoots, (poke), raw	202.7	338
Peppers, sweet, green, sautéed	203.6	339
Currants, European black, raw	202.7	338
Kiwifruit, gold, raw	196	327
Mustard spinach, (tendergreen), raw	195	325
Peppers, sweet, red, raw	190.3	317
Apple juice, frozen concentrate, unsweetened, undiluted, with added ascorbic acid	187.6	313
Peppers, sweet, red, sautéed	172.6	288
Tomato juice, canned, with salt added	170.3	284
Kiwifruit, green, raw	166.9	278
Drumstick pods, raw	141	235

Source: U.S. Department of Agriculture, Agricultural Research Service (2015). USDA National Nutrient Database for Standard Reference, Release 27.

and oxalic acid. However, when large doses (2 g/day) of vitamin C are consumed, it may be excreted unchanged as ascorbic acid.

In our bodies, vitamin C acts as an antioxidant or reducing agent. Extra electrons present in the vitamin C molecule may be donated to free radicals, therefore reducing them. This is commonly referred to as "quenching" free radicals. Free radicals are naturally produced by oxidative processes in the body, but when left unquenched, they may lead to a destructive cascade resulting in damage to or death of healthy cells. Ascorbic acid is also necessary for the healthy production of collagen through its ability to maintain iron in its reduced state, which is necessary for the proper function of the collagen producing enzyme, proline monooxygenase. Collagen is an important component of connective tissues such as skin, tendons, ligaments, cartilage, bone, and blood vessels, and by weight, and it is the most abundant protein found in the body. Vitamin C is also required for the synthesis of hormones including melanotropin, norepinephrine, and epinephrine. Ascorbic acid also plays several key roles in immune function. Vitamin C stimulates the production and function of leukocytes, namely neutrophils, lymphocytes, and phagocytes (Anderson et al. 1980). Vitamin C also stimulates cellular motility, chemotaxis, and phagocytosis, all functions essential to optimal performance of the immune system. Vitamin C has also been demonstrated to increase the levels of antibodies and complement proteins, important players in immune function (Anderson et al. 1980). As an antioxidant, vitamin C also protects the integrity of immune cells that are under constant attack by free radicals created in the immune process (Jariwalla and Harakeh 1996, 1997). Supplementation of high doses of vitamin C (60 mg/kg body weight) have also been shown to increase NK cell activity up to 10-fold (Heuser and Vojdani 1997).

Vitamin C is found in the body in three forms, ascorbic acid, semidehydroascorbic acid, and dehydroascorbic acid. Conversion of free radicals to stable molecules takes vitamin C through these stages. Removal of one electron creates semidehydroascorbic acid, or the ascorbate radical. The removal of the second electron creates dehydroascorbate (Brody 1999). Dehydroascorbate is regenerated into ascorbic acid via the enzyme dehydroascorbate reductase, and this process requires the endogenous antioxidant glutathione.

Rationale for Supplementation

The DV for vitamin C is currently set at 60 mg for adults and children, age four and older. The National Health and Nutrition Examination

Survey (NHANES) from 2001 to 2002 found that mean intakes of vitamin C were ~105.2 mg/day for adult males and 83.6 mg/day for adult females, which exceeds the DV (Mosfegh, Goldman, and Cleveland 2005). Despite adequate intake levels of vitamin C from the diet, vitamin C dietary supplement use is common. Approximately 12 percent of adults in the United States take a vitamin C supplement (Radimer et al. 2004).

The most common health benefit attributed to Vitamin C is immune support. A Cochrane review of vitamin C use for the common cold was published in 2007 (Douglas et al. 2007). This meta-analysis found that, in adults and in children, regular vitamin C supplementation resulted in a significant reduction in the duration of respiratory episodes that occurred during the long-term supplementation period, although results of therapeutic trials were not significant. Most immunity-targeted supplements contain high doses of vitamin C and most vitamin C supplements claim immune support as their key benefit.

Another common motive for vitamin C supplementation is its support of healthy connective tissues found in cartilage, tendons, ligaments, bone, skin, and blood vessels. Vitamin C supports healthy collagen formation, and collagen is an important component of these connective tissues. Vitamin C supplementation in conjunction with estrogen in postmenopausal women was found to support healthy bone mineral density. This benefit is an important factor in wound healing.

CV benefits of vitamin C supplementation have also been studied, with conflicting results. A clinical trial of 1,000 mg/day vitamin C supplementation resulted in a decrease in low-density lipoprotein (LDL) cholesterol and an increase in healthy high-density lipoprotein (HDL) cholesterol (Gatto et al. 1996), while a similar study found no CV benefit (Jacques et al. 1995). In nonsmoking individuals exposed to smoke in the air, 3 g of vitamin C per day prevented smoke-induced decreases in plasma antioxidant defenses, the resistance of LDL cholesterol to oxidation and reactive substances called thiobarbituric acid reactive substances (TBARS), which are formed as a byproduct of lipid peroxidation (Valkonen and Kuusi 2000). This data suggests possible CV benefits may be a result of vitamin C supplementation, furthermore, results suggest that baseline vitamin C levels may affect the likelihood of a benefit from supplementation.

Safety

As a water-soluble vitamin, severe toxicity associated with vitamin C intake is rare, and consumption at levels less than 5 g/day is generally seen as safe (Diplock et al. 1998; Pearce, Boosalis, and Yeager 2000). In some individuals, osmotic diarrhea may occur with bolus doses greater than 1 g/d, and this symptom may be occasionally accompanied by fatigue, insomnia, or headache, but these symptoms appear to be transient.

Speculation around a link between high doses of vitamin C and kidney stones exists, but has not been supported by clinical evidence. While oxalate, the chief component of kidney stones, is a byproduct of ascorbic acid metabolism, its plasma levels have not been found to be affected by vitamin C supplementation. Oxalate excretion does not appear to be dose-dependently affected by vitamin C supplementation, and an association between vitamin C supplementation and kidney stone prevalence is not apparent (Garewal and Diplock 1995; Simon and Hudes 1999).

Finally, some concern lies around a possible pro-oxidant effect of large supplemented doses of vitamin C. Research in this area shows that the concerns may be warranted, but the topic is highly controversial (Halliwell 1996). In vitro studies suggest that interactions of vitamin C with metal ions may contribute to oxidative damage (Primack 1999) However, in vivo studies challenge this data as vitamin C in biologic fluids, animals, and humans was found to provide antioxidant protection of lipids even in the presence of metal ions (Carr and Frei 1999).

B Vitamins

Background

There are eight vitamins that make up the B-Vitamin complex including thiamin (vitamin B1), riboflavin (vitamin B2), niacin (vitamin B3), pyridoxine (vitamin B6), folate, cyanocobalamin (vitamin B12), pantothenic acid, and biotin. These vitamins are water soluble, meaning they solubilize in water, are not stored in the body, and excess amounts ingested are secreted in the urine. Sufficient levels of B vitamins are not stored in the body; therefore, regular intake of these vitamins from dietary sources is necessary. They are often found together in foods and have similar coenzyme functions, often requiring the presence of one or more of the others for optimal performance. For example, the enzyme pyruvate dehydrogenase requires the presence of riboflavin, thiamin, niacin and pantothenic acid, four of the B vitamins, for optimal function. Intestinal bacteria are capable of producing some of the B vitamins, but the majority of the required amounts of these nutrients are acquired from the diet. Some foods, including refined flour products, sugar, coffee, and alcohol can deplete B vitamins. As intakes of these foods increase, as is common in the western diet, requirements for the B vitamins also increase.

There are two categories of B-vitamins—those involved in the chemical reactions used to create energy by the body and those used to transfer single-carbon units throughout the body. The former group consists of thiamin, riboflavin, niacin, vitamin B6, and pantothenic acid, with the remainder making up the single-carbon group transfer cluster.

Thiamin, also known as vitamin B1 is the first of the B vitamins. The RDA for thiamin is 1.5 mg/day. Thiamin is present in a variety of foods both of plant and animal origin, as well as in yeast. When consumed in food, the cofactor form of thiamin, thiamin pyrophosphate (TPP) is released from dietary proteins and then hydrolyzed into thiamin during the digestive process. The thiamin is absorbed into the blood stream and transported to various tissues, where it is converted back into TPP by the enzyme thiaminokinase. Thiamin pyrophosphate is a cofactor for the enzymes pyruvate dehydrogenase, alpha-ketoglutarate dehydrogenase, and branched chain keto acid (BCKA) dehydrogenase, which catalyze the reduction of nicotinamide adenine dinucleotide (NAD) and transketolase, which catalyzes the transfer of 2-carbon units at two places of the pentose phosphate pathway. NAD is an electron acceptor in the energy producing pathways for the breakdown of carbohydrates, fatty acids, ketone bodies, amino acids, and alcohol. The pentose-phosphate pathway is responsible for the metabolism of some sugars and the synthesis of ribose-5-phosphate, a key component of the nucleic acids including ATP, the body's cellular energy substrate (Brody 1999).

A severe deficiency in thiamin intake results in the disease beriberi. Symptoms of beriberi include difficulty in walking, loss of feeling in the hands and feet, loss of muscle function or paralysis of the lower legs, mental confusion and speech difficulties, pain, strange eye movements, tingling, and vomiting. For individuals suffering from beriberi associated with alcoholism, also classified as wet beriberi, symptoms include awakening at night short of breath, increased heart rate, shortness of breath with activity, and swelling of the lower legs.

Riboflavin, or vitamin B2 is the second B vitamin. The RDA for riboflavin is 1.7 mg/day. Liver is the most abundant source of riboflavin, but it is also found in meat, dairy products, dark green vegetables, grains, and legumes. After consumption and digestion of foods containing riboflavin, it is absorbed by the gut, mainly in the ileum and enters the bloodstream. During the absorption process, or postabsorption in the organs, riboflavin is converted to its cofactor Flavin mononucleotide (FMN) by the enzyme flavokinase and then to Flavin adenine dinucleotide (FAD) by FAD synthase. These flavins are cofactors for a large number of enzymes (about 50), most notably dihydrolipoyl dehydrogenase, a component of pyruvate dehydrogenase and alpha-ketoglutarate dehydrogenase, fatty acyl-CoA dehydrogenase, succinate dehydrogenase, and NADH dehydrogenase, which are used in energy metabolism pathways. The FAD portions of these enzymes accept and transfer electrons through these pathways (Brody 1999). Riboflavin deficiency causes lesions of the mouth known as cheilosis and angular stomatitis, but is extremely rare.

Niacin, or vitamin B3, is the third B vitamin. The RDA for niacin is 19 mg for adult men and 14 mg for adult women. Niacin is found in many foods, but most abundantly in meat, eggs, fish, dairy products, and whole wheat. In food, niacin occurs mainly as NAD or NADP (the phosphorylated form NAD). In the gut, NAD and NADP are hydrolyzed by enzymes into nicotinamide or nicotinamide nucleotide. These molecules are broken down by enzymes in the liver and gut into nicotinic acid. In the body, nicotinic acid is then converted back to NAD. The role of NAD in energy metabolism has been discussed earlier in this chapter. NAD is also used in posttranslational modification of proteins on human chromosomes that help support the helical structure of DNA, and help regulate gene expression. NAD also serves as a substrate for

Poly (ADP-ribose) polymerase, an enzyme important for cell growth, cell differentiation, and DNA repair (Satoh, Poirier, and Lindahl 1993). Nutritional deficiency of niacin is called pellagra. Symptoms of pellagra include severe dermatitis and fissured scabs, diarrhea, and mental depression.

Pyridoxine is vitamin B6, the fourth B vitamin. The RDA for pyridoxine is 2.0 mg for adults. Good dietary sources of vitamin B6 include poultry, fish, liver, and eggs and to a lesser extent, meat and milk. Vitamin B6 in plants such as beans, carrots, orange juice, and broccoli is found primarily as pyridoxine glucoside. This format is less bioavailable than the form found in animal foods. Vitamin B6 is released from food and absorbed in the intestine via saturable transporters. Once absorbed, the pyridoxine is converted into the bioactive forms of pyridoxal 5'-phosphate (PLP) and pyridoxamine phosphate (PMP) in the liver. PLP is the cofactor for a large number of enzymes used in amino acid metabolism. Vitamin B6 deficiency is most common in alcoholics due to a combination of low intake of the vitamin and alcohol-induced impairment of vitamin B6 metabolism. Symptoms of vitamin B6 deficiency include depression, confusion, and occasional convulsions. Vitamin B6 may be toxic at doses 1,000 times the RDA. Daily intake of 2 to 5 g of vitamin B6 can result in difficulty walking and in tingling sensations in legs and soles of the feet. These conditions may be reversed if toxic doses are discontinued.

Folate is the fifth B vitamin. The RDA for folate is 200 mcg/day for adult men and 180 mcg/day for adult women. Folate is essential for the healthy development of an embryo, and therefore, RDAs are increased during pregnancy to 400 mcg/day. Liver, egg yolk, orange juice, and green vegetables are good sources of folate. In dietary supplements, folate is most commonly provided as folic acid, however this is not the most common form in which the vitamin is found in nature. The folic acid form of folate is easily absorbed and converted to the active forms, dihydrofolate and tetrahydrofolate, in most people; however, there are some individuals with genetic polymorphisms that inhibit this ability, and these individuals must take the active form of the vitamin, methyltetrahydrofolate. In the gut, gamma-glutamyl hydrolase is required for the absorption of folic acid. Once absorbed, dietary folate is taken up into the blood in the mono-glutamyl form, t-methyl-H_4folylmonoglutamate.

The folate is transported into cells in this form, where it is converted to the polygutamyl form by folylpolyglutamate synthase. This format helps keep the folate in the cell and enhances its ability to bind to folate-requiring enzymes and the ability of folate to shuttle from one active site on an enzyme to another without dissociating (Brody 1999; Paquin, Baugh, and MacKenzie 1985). Folate is a cofactor in 1-carbon metabolism reactions in the methylation cycle. In this cycle, methionine synthase catalyses the transfer of a 1-carbon unit from folate to homocysteine, creating methionine. Methionine is then converted to S-adenosylmethionine (SAM), a universal methyl donor for close to 100 different substrates including DNA, RNA, hormones, proteins, and lipids. Donation of the methyl group converts SAM to S-adenosylhomocysteine, which is broken down into homocysteine, completing the methylation cycle. Folate is also required for the formation of purines and pyrimidines (Brody 1999).

Cobalamin is vitamin B12, the sixth B vitamin. The RDA for vitamin B12 is 2.0 mcg/day for adult men and women. Vitamin B12 is found in animal products, but is not present in plant products. Therefore, vitamin B12 deficiency is a common concern for individuals consuming strict vegetarian or vegan diets. Vitamin B12 is the largest and most complex of all of the vitamins, and it contains the metal ion cobalt. In food, vitamin B12 is usually bound to protein, and is released by the activity of hydrochloric acid and gastric protease in the stomach (Board 1998). Synthetic vitamin B12 does not require this step as it is already in the free form. Once freed, vitamin B12 combines with intrinsic factor and is absorbed in the distal ileum by receptor-mediated endocytosis. The active form of vitamin B12 in the body is methylcobalamin. In the body, vitamin B12 is required for proper red blood cell formation, neurological function, and DNA synthesis. Methylcobalamin is a cofactor for methionine synthase and L-methylmalonyl-CoA mutase. The process of methionine synthase in the methylation cycle has been described earlier. L-methylmalonyl-CoA mutase is an enzyme that converts L-methylmalonyl-CoA to succinyl-CoA in the degradation of propionate, an essential reaction in fat and protein metabolism (Combs 1992). Vitamin B12 deficiency is characterized by megaloblastic anemia, fatigue, weakness, constipation, loss of appetite, weight loss, numbness and tingling in the hands and feet, compromised balance, depression, confusion, dementia, poor memory, and soreness of the mouth or tongue. Large amounts of folic acid can mask vitamin B12 deficiency as it corrects the most common symptom, megaloblastic anemia.

Pantothenic acid is the seventh B vitamin. There is no RDA for pantothenic acid as it is present in all plant and animal foods. The richest sources of pantothenic acid are liver, yeast, egg yolk, and vegetables. In food, pantothenic acid is found as coenzyme A. In the gut, coenzyme A is hydrolyzed into pantothenic acid, which is easily absorbed. Pantothenic acid is then carried through the bloodstream to various tissues, where it is converted back to coenzyme A. Coenzyme A is used in the Krebs cycle, fatty acid synthesis and oxidation, amino acid metabolism, ketone body metabolism, cholesterol synthesis, and conjugation of bile salts. Pantothenic acid deficiency does not occur naturally, except in those with severe malnutrition.

Biotin is the eighth and final B vitamin. Like pantothenic acid, there is no RDA for Biotin, as it is produced by the gut microflora. Biotin is also found naturally in milk. Biotin is a cofactor for five carboxylases, acetyl-CoA carboxylase, pyruvate carboxylase, propionyl-CoA carboxylase, 3-methylcrotonyl-CoA carboxylase, and geranyl-CoA carboxylase. As a part of these enzymes, biotin plays an essential role in fatty acid metabolism, amino acid metabolism, carbohydrate metabolism, polyketide biosynthesis, urea utilization, and other cellular processes (Tong 2013). Biotin deficiency associated with decreased dietary intake is rare.

Rationale for Supplementation

B vitamin complex products are most commonly taken by consumers for energy support. Common marketing claims used on B vitamin complex labels include "provides energy support," "vitality," and "supports energy production." These claims are permitted on products providing a variety of B vitamins due to the role that B vitamins play in the metabolism of food and the resulting production of energy. However, these products, when they contain only B vitamins, do not produce stimulant-like effects on physical energy levels; so consumers should not expect these outcomes with supplementation.

Similar to multivitamins, some consumers may also turn to B vitamin "complex" products as a supplement to their dietary intake, to fill possible gaps in their daily consumption of these vitamins. The U.S. NHANES study results from 2003 to 2008 have found that dieters' surveys indicate below average vitamin intake in Western countries depending on fortification levels of food, local dietary habits, and socioeconomic status. They found that 5 to 50 percent of men and women consume the B vitamins thiamin, riboflavin, niacin, B6, B12, and folic acid below the recommended intakes (Troesch et al. 2012). Therefore, a B vitamin complex product may be beneficial for these individuals.

Some of the individual B vitamins are also marketed for the specific health benefits associated with those nutrients, including niacin for CV support, folate for prenatal health, and vitamin B12 to support a deficient vegetarian diet. These products are usually marketed as single ingredients, rather than as a complex of all of the B vitamins together.

Safety

B vitamins are likely safe when taken orally at recommended dosages. TULs have not been determined for thiamin, riboflavin, vitamin B12, pantothenic acid, or biotin. A lack of suitable studies at extremely high levels prevents reliable estimates of upper levels that can be ingested safely. TULs have been developed for niacin (35 mg/day), vitamin B6 (100 mg/day), and folate (1,000 mg/day) in an effort to protect the most vulnerable individuals in the general population (Board 1998). Consumption of B complex products containing levels of these vitamins in excess of the TULs for extended periods of time are not recommended.

References

Abrams, S.A. 2010. "Setting Dietary Reference Intakes with the Use of Bioavailability Data: Calcium." *American Journal of Clinical Nutrition* 91, no. 5, pp. 1474S–77S. doi:10.3945/ajcn.2010.28674H

Alvir, J.M., and S. Thys-Jacobs. 1991. "Premenstrual and Menstrual Symptom Clusters and Response to Calcium Treatment." *Psychopharmacology Bulletin* 27, no. 2, pp. 145–48.

Anderson, J.J., and P.J. Klemmer. 2013. "Risk of High Dietary Calcium for Arterial Calcification in Older Adults." *Nutrients* 5, no. 10, pp. 3964–74. doi:10.3390/nu5103964.

Anderson, J.L., H.T. May, B.D. Horne, T.L. Bair, N.L. Hall, J.F. Carlquist, D.L. Lappé, and J.B. Muhlestein. 2010. "Relation of Vitamin D Deficiency to Cardiovascular Risk Factors, Disease Status, and Incident Events in a General Healthcare Population." *The American Journal of Cardiology* 106, no. 7, pp. 963–68. doi:10.1016/j.amjcard.2010.05.027

Anderson, R., R. Oosthuizen, R. Maritz, A. Theron, and A.J. Van Rensburg. 1980. "The Effects of Increasing Weekly Doses of Ascorbate on certain Cellular and Humoral Immune Functions in Normal Volunteers." *The American Journal of Clinical Nutrition* 33, no. 1, pp. 71–76.

Bailey, R.L. 2015. "Multivitamin-Mineral Use Is Associated with Reduced Risk of Cardiovascular Disease Mortality among Women in the United States." *Journal of Nutrition* 145, no. 3, pp. 572–78. doi:10.3945/jn.114.204743

Bender, D.A. 2003. *Nutritional Biochemistry of the Vitamins*. 2nd ed. Cambridge, UK: Cambridge University Press.

Bertone-Johnson, E.R., S.E. Hankinson, A. Bendich, S.R. Johnson, W.C. Willett, and J.E. Manson. 2005. "Calcium and Vitamin D intake and Risk of Incident Premenstrual Syndrome." *Archives of Internal Medicine* 165, no. 11, pp. 1246–52. doi:10.1001/archinte.165.11.1246

Bouillon, R., G. Carmeliet, L. Verlinden, E. van Etten, A. Verstuyf, H.F. Luderer, L. Lieben, C. Mathieu, and M. Demay. 2008. "Vitamin D and Human Health: Lessons from Vitamin D Receptor Null Mice." *Endocrine Reviews* 29, no. 6, pp. 726–76. doi:10.1210/er.2008-0004

Bradley, J.S., R.T. Wassel, L. Lee, and S. Nambiar. 2009. "Intravenous Ceftriaxone and Calcium in the Neonate: Assessing the Risk for Cardiopulmonary Adverse Events." *Pediatrics* 123, no. 4. pp. 609–13. doi:10.1542/peds.2008-3080

Brody, T. 1999. *Nutritional Biochemistry*. 2nd ed. San Diego, CA: Academic Press.

Bryant, R.J., J. Cadogan, and C.M. Weaver. 1999. "The New Dietary Reference Intakes for Calcium: Implications for Osteoporosis." *Journal of American College Nutrition* 18, no. 5 Suppl, pp. 406S–412S. doi:10.1080/07315724. 1999.10718905

Calcium Professional Monograph. Available from https://naturalmedicines. therapeuticresearch.com/databases/food,-herbs-supplements/professional. aspx?productid=781.

Carr, A., and B. Frei. 1999. "Does Vitamin C Act as a Pro-Oxidant under Physiological Conditions?" *FASEB Journal* 13, no. 9, pp. 1007–24. doi:10.1096/fj.1530-6860

Carroll, C., K. Cooper, D. Papaioannou, D. Hind, H. Pilgrim, and P. Tappenden. 2010. "Supplemental Calcium in the Chemoprevention of Colorectal Cancer: A Systematic Review and Meta-Analysis." *Clinical Therapeutics* 32, no. 5, pp. 789–803. doi:10.1016/j.clinthera.2010.04.024

Chiu, K.M. 1999. "Efficacy of Calcium Supplements on Bone Mass in Postmenopausal Women." *The Journals of Gerontology Series A: Biological Sciences and Medical Sciences* 54, no. 6, pp. M275–80. doi:10.1093/gerona/54.6.m275

Combs, G. 1992. *Vitamins B12 in The Vitamins.* New York: Academic Press, Inc.

Cooper, K., H. Squires, C. Carroll, D. Papaioannou, A. Booth, R.F. Logan, C. Maguire, D. Hind, and P. Tappenden. 2010. "Chemoprevention of Colorectal Cancer: Systematic Review and Economic Evaluation." *Health Technology Assessment* 14, no. 32, pp. 1–206. doi:10.3310/hta14320

Cumming, R.G., and M.C. Nevitt. 1997. "Calcium for Prevention of Osteoporotic Fractures in Postmenopausal Women." *Journal Bone Mineral Research* 12, no. 9, pp. 1321–29. doi:10.1359/jbmr.1997.12.9.1321

Diplock, A.T., J.L. Charleux, G. Crozier-Willi, F.J. Kok, C. Rice-Evans, M. Roberfroid, W. Stahl, and J. Vina-Ribes. 1998. "Functional Food Science and Defence Against Reactive Oxidative Species." *British Journal of Nutrition* 80 Suppl 1, pp. S77–112. doi:10.1079/bjn19980106

Dobnig, H., S. Pilz, H. Scharnagl, W. Renner, U. Seelhorst, B. Wellnitz, J. Kinkeldei, B.O. Boehm, G. Weihrauch, and W. Maerz. 2008. " Independent Association of Low Serum 25-Hydroxyvitamin D and 1,25-Dihydroxyvitamin D Levels with All-Cause and Cardiovascular Mortality." *Archives of Internal Medicine* pp. 1340–49. doi:10.1001/archinte.168.12.1340

Douglas, R.M., H. Hemila, E. Chalker, and B. Treacy. 2007. "Vitamin C for Preventing and Treating the Common Cold." *Cochrane Database of Systematic Reviews* no. 3, pp. CD000980. doi:10.1002/14651858.CD000980.pub3

Food and Nutrition Board of the Institute of Medicine. 1998. *Dietary Reference Intakes: Thiamin, Riboflavin, Niacin, Vitamin B6, Folate, Vitamin B12, Pantothenic Acid, Biotin, and Choline.* Washington, DC: National Academy Press.

Forman, J.P., J.B. Scott, K. Ng, B.F. Drake, E.G. Suarez, D.L. Hayden, G.G. Bennett, P.D. Chandler, B.W. Hollis, K.M. Emmons, E.L. Giovannucci, C.S. Fuchs, and A.T. Chan. 2013. "Effect of Vitamin D Supplementation on Blood Pressure in Blacks." *Hypertension* 61, no. 4, pp. 779–85. doi:10.1161/hypertensionaha.111.00659

Gahche, J., R. Bailey, V. Burt, J. Hughes, E. Yetley, J. Dwyer, M.F. Picciano, M. McDowell, and C. Sempos. 2011. "Dietary Supplement Use Among U.S. Adults Has Increased Since NHANES III (1988–1994)." *NCHS Data Brief* no. 61, Hyattsville, MD: National Center for Health Statistics.

Garewal, H.S., and A.T. Diplock. 1995. "How 'Safe' Are Antioxidant Vitamins?" *Drug Safety* 13, 1, pp. 8–14. doi:10.2165/00002018-199513010-00002

Gatto, L.M., G.K. Hallen, A.J. Brown, and S. Samman. 1996. "Ascorbic Acid Induces a Favorable Lipoprotein Profile in Women." *Journal of the American College of Nutrition* 15, no. 2, pp. 154–8. doi:10.1080/07315724.1996.107 18581

Gunta, S.S., R.I. Thadhani, and R.H. Mak. 2013. "The Effect of Vitamin D Status on Risk Factors for Cardiovascular Disease." *Nature Review Nephrology* 9, no. 6, pp. 337–47. doi:/10.1038/nrneph.2013.74

Halliwell, B. 1996. "Vitamin C: Antioxidant or Pro-Oxidant in Vivo?" *Free Radical Research* 25, no. 5, pp. 439–54. doi:10.3109/10715769609149066

Heuser, G., and A. Vojdani. 1997. "Enhancement of Natural Killer Cell Activity and T and B Cell Function by Buffered Vitamin C in Patients Exposed to Toxic Chemicals: The Role of Protein Kinase-C." *Immunopharmacology Immunotoxicology* 19, no. 3, pp. 291–312. doi:10.3109/08923979709046977.

Holick, M.F. 2007. "Vitamin D Deficiency." *The New England Journal of Medicine* 357, no. 3, pp. 266–81. doi:10.1056/NEJMra070553

Huang, H-Y., B. Caballero, S. Chang, A.J. Alberg, R.D. Semba, C. Schneyer, R.F. Wilson, T-Y. Cheng, G. Prokopowicz, G.J. Barnes II, J. Vassy, and E.B. Bass. 2006. *Multivitamin/Mineral Supplements and Prevention of Chronic Disease.* Evidence Report/Technology Assessment. Rockville, MD: Agency for Healthcare Research and Quality.

Institute of Medicine (U.S.) Standing Committee on the Scientific Evaluation of Dietary Reference Intakes. 1997. *Dietary Reference Intakes for Calcium, Phosphorus, Magnesium, Vitamin D, and Fluoride.* Washington, DC: National Academy Press.

Jacques, P.F., S.I. Sulsky, G.E. Perrone, J. Jenner, and E.J. Schaefer. 1995. "Effect of Vitamin C Supplementation on Lipoprotein Cholesterol, Apolipoprotein, and Triglyceride Concentrations." *Annals of Epidemiology* 5, no. 1, pp. 52–9. doi:10.1016/1047-2797(94)00041-q

Jariwalla, R.J., and S. Harakeh. 1996. "Antiviral and Immunomodulatory Activities of Ascorbic Acid." In *Subcellular Biochemistry. Ascorbic Acid: Biochemistry and Biomedical Cell Biology*, edited by J.R. Harris, 215–31. New York: Plenum Press.

Jariwalla, R.J., and S. Harakeh. 1997. "Mechanisms Underlying the Action of Vitamin C in Viral and Immunodeficiency Disease." In *Vitamin C in Health and Disease.*, eds. L. Packer and J. Fuchs, 309–22. New York: Marcel Dekker Inc.

Kienreich, K., A. Tomaschitz, N. Verheyen, T. Pieber, M. Gaksch, M.R. Grübler, and S. Pilz. 2013. "Vitamin D and Cardiovascular Disease." *Nutrients* 5, no. 8, pp. 3005–21. doi:10.3390/nu5083005

Ku, Y.C., M.E. Liu, C.S. Ku, T.Y. Liu, and S.L. Lin. 2013. "Relationship Between Vitamin D Deficiency and Cardiovascular Disease." *World Journal Cardiology* 5, no. 9, pp. 337–46. doi:10.4330/wjc.v5.i9.337

Kunutsor, S.K., T.A. Apekey, and M. Steur. 2013. "Vitamin D and Risk of Future Hypertension: Meta-Analysis of 283,537 Participants." *European Journal of Epidemiology* 28, no. 3, pp. 205–21. doi:10.1007/s10654-013-9790-2

Larsen, T., F.H. Mose, J.N. Bech, A.B. Hansen, and E.B. Pedersen. 2012. "Effect of Cholecalciferol Supplementation During Winter Months in Patients with Hypertension: A Randomized, Placebo-Controlled Trial." *American Journal of Hypertension* 25, no. 11, pp. 1215–22. doi:10.1038/ajh.2012.111

Lawson, K.A., M.E. Wright, A. Subar, T. Mouw, A. Hollenbeck, A. Schatzkin, and M.F. Leitzmann. 2007. "Multivitamin Use and Risk of Prostate Cancer in the National Institutes of Health-AARP Diet and Health Study." *Journal of the National Cancer Institute* 99, no. 10, pp. 754–64. doi:10.1093/jnci/djk177

Li, Y.C., J. Kong, M. Wei, Z.F. Chen, S.Q. Liu, L.P. Cao. 2002. "1,25-Dihydroxyvitamin D(3) is a Negative Endocrine Regulator of the Renin-Angiotensin System." *Journal of Clinical Investion* 110, no. 2, pp. 229–38. doi:10.1172/jci15219

Maton, P.N., and M.E. Burton. 1999. "Antacids Revisited: A Review of Their Clinical Pharmacology and Recommended Therapeutic Use." *Drugs* 57, no. 6, pp. 855–70. doi:10.2165/00003495-199957060-00003

McGreevy, C., and D. Williams. 2011. "New Insights About Vitamin D and Cardiovascular Disease: A Narrative Review." *Annals of Internal Medicine* 155, no. 12, pp. 820–26.

Mendall, M.A., P. Patel M. Asante, L. Ballam, J. Morris, D.P. Strachan, A.J. Camm, and T.C. 1997. Northfield. Relation of Serum Cytokine Concentrations to Cardiovascular Risk Factors and Coronary Heart Disease. *Heart* 78, no. 3, pp. 273–77.

Michos, E.D., and M.L. Melamed. 2008. "Vitamin D and Cardiovascular Disease Risk." *Current Opinion in Clinical Nutrition and Metabolic Care* 11, no. 1, pp. 7–12. doi:10.1097/MCO.0b013e3282f2f4dd

Mithal, A., On behalf of the IOF Committee of Scientific Advisors (CSA) Nutrition Working Group, D.A. Wahl, J.-P. Bonjour, P. Burckhardt, B. Dawson-Hughes, J.A. Eisman, G. El-Hajj Fuleihan, R.G. Josse, P. Lips, and J. Morales-Torres. 2009. "Global Vitamin D Status and Determinants of Hypovitaminosis D." *Osteoporosis. International* 20, no. 11, pp. 1807–20. doi:10.1007/s00198-009-0954-6

Mosfegh, A., J. Goldman, and L. Cleveland. 2005. *What We Eat in America*, NHANES 2001–2002: Usual Nutrient Intakes from Food Compared to Dietary References Intakes. Washington, DC: U.S. Department of Agriculture, Agricultural Research Service.

Muth, M.K., D.W. Anderson, J.L. Domanico, J.B Smith, and B. Wendling. 1999. Economic Characterization of the Dietary Supplement Industry. Final, Research Triangle Park, NC: Research Triangle Institute.

Nathanson, M.H. 1994. "Cellular and Subcellular Calcium Signaling in Gastrointestinal Epithelium." Gastroenterology 106, no. 5, pp. 1349–64.

National Osteoporosis Foundation. 2010. 2010 Clinician's Guide to Prevention and Treatment of Osteoporosis. www.nof.org/sites/default/files/pdfs/NOF_ClinicianGuide2009_v7.pdf

Natural Medicines Database. Available from https://naturalmedicines.therapeuticresearch.com/

Nieves, J.W., L. Komar, F. Cosman, and R. Lindsay. 1998. "Calcium Potentiates the Effect of Estrogen and Calcitonin on Bone Mass: Review and Analysis." American Journal of Clinical Nutrition 67, no. 1, pp. 18–24.

NIH, Office of Dietary Supplements. July 2015. Multivitamin/mineral Supplements Fact Sheet for Health Professionals. https://ods.od.nih.gov/factsheets/MVMS-HealthProfessional/ (accessed July 10, 2015).

NIH, State-of-the-Science Panel. 2007. "National Institutes of Health State-of-the-Science Conference Statement: Multivitamin/Mineral Supplements and Chronic Disease Prevention." American Journal Clinical Nutrition 85, no. 1, pp. 257S–64S.

Nordin, B.E. 2009. "The Effect of Calcium Supplementation on Bone Loss in 32 Controlled Trials in Postmenopausal Women." Osteoporosis International 20, no. 12, pp. 2135–43. doi:10.1007/s00198-009-0926-x

NPCS Board. 2012. Detailed Project Profiles on Chemical Industries Vol II. 2nd Revised Ed. New Delhi, India: NIIR PROJECT CONSULTANCY SERVICES.

Paquin, J., C.M. Baugh, and R.E. MacKenzie. 1985. "Channeling Between the Active Sites of Formiminotransferase-Cyclodeaminase. Binding and Kinetic Studies." Journal of Biological Chemistry 260, no. 28, pp. 14925–31.

Pearce, K.A., M.G. Boosalis, and B. Yeager. 2000. "Update on Vitamin Supplements for the Prevention of Coronary Disease and Stroke." American Family Physician 62, no. 6, pp. 1359–66.

Penland, J.G., and P.E. Johnson. 1993. "Dietary Calcium and Manganese Effects on Menstrual Cycle Symptoms." American Journal of Obstetrics and Gynecology 168, no. 5, pp. 1417–23. doi:10.1016/s0002-9378(11)90775-3

Pennington, J.A., and S.A. Schoen. 1996. "Total Diet Study: Estimated Dietary Intakes of Nutritional Elements, 1982–1991." International Journal for Vitamin and Nutrition Research 66, no. 4, pp. 350–62.

Primack, A. 1999. "Complementary/Alternative Therapies in the Prevention and Treatment of Cancer." In Complementary/Alternative Medicine: An Evidence-Based Approach, eds. J.W. Spencer and J.J. Jacobs. St. Louis, MO: Mosby.

Radimer, K., B. Bindewald, J. Hughes, B. Ervin, C. Swanson, and M.F. Picciano. 2004. "Dietary Supplement use by US Adults: Data from the National Health and Nutrition Examination Survey, 1999-2000." *American Journal of Epidemiology* 160, no. 4, pp. 339–49. doi:10.1093/aje/kwh207

Ramagopalan, S.V., A. Heger, A.J. Berlanga, N.J. Maugeri, M.R. Lincoln, A. Burrell, L. Handunnetthi, A.E. Handel, G. Disanto, S.-M. Orton, C.T. Watson, J.M. Morahan, G. Giovannoni, C.P. Ponting, G.C. Ebers, and J.C. Knight. 2010. "A ChIP-seq Defined Genome-wide Map of Vitamin D Receptor Binding: Associations with Disease and Evolution." *Genome Research* 20, no. 10, pp. 1352–60. doi:10.3410/f.10050958.10802057

Rasmussen, H. 1986. "The Calcium Messenger System (2)." *The New England Journal of Medicine* 314, no. 18, pp. 1164–70. doi:10.1056/NEJM198605013141807

Rostand, S.G., and T.B. Drüeke. 1999. "Parathyroid Hormone, Vitamin D, and Cardiovascular Disease in Chronic Renal Failure." *Kidney International* 56, no. 2, pp. 383–92. doi:10.1046/j.1523-1755.1999.00575.x

Satoh, M.S., G.G. Poirier, and T. Lindahl. 1993. "NAD(+)-Dependent Repair of Damaged DNA by Human Cell Extracts." *Journal of Biological Chemistry* 268, no. 8, pp. 5480–87.

Savini, I., A. Rossi, C. Pierro, L. Avigliano, and M.V. Catani. 2008. "SVCT1 and SVCT2: Key Proteins for Vitamin C Uptake." *Amino Acids* 34, no. 3, pp. 347–55. doi:10.1007/s00726-007-0555-7

Shearman, D.J. 1978. "Vitamin A and Sir Douglas Mawson." *BMJ* 1, no. 6108, pp. 283–85. doi:10.1136/bmj.1.6108.283

Simon, J.A., and E.S. Hudes. 1999. "Relation of Serum Ascorbic Acid to Serum Vitamin B12, Serum Ferritin, and Kidney Stones in US Adults." *Archives of Internal Medicine* 159, no. 6, pp. 619–24. doi:10.1001/archinte.159.6.619

Stewart, A.F., and A.E. Broadus. 1987. "Mineral Metabolism." In *Endocrinology and Metabolism*, eds. P. Felig, J.D. Baxter, A.E. Broadus and L.A. Frohman, 1317. New York: McGraw-Hill.

Sullivan, G.W., I.J. Sarembock, and J. Linden. 2000. "The Role of Inflammation in Vascular Diseases." *Journal of Leukocyte Biology* 67, no. 5, pp. 591–602.

Thys-Jacobs, S., P. Starkey, D. Bernstein, and J. Tian. 1998. "Calcium Carbonate and the Premenstrual Syndrome: Effects on Premenstrual and Menstrual Symptoms. Premenstrual Syndrome Study Group." *American Journal of Obstetrics andGynecology* 179, no. 2, pp. 444–52. doi:10.1016/s0002-9378(98)70377-1

Tong, L. 2013. "Structure and Function of Biotin-Dependent Carboxylases." *Cellular and Molecular Life Sciences* 70, no. 5, pp. 863–91. doi:10.1007/s00018-012-1096-0

Troesch, B., B. Hoeft, M. McBurney, M. Eggersdorfer, and P. Weber. 2012. "Dietary Surveys Indicate Vitamin Intakes Below Recommendations are Common in Representative Western Countries." *British Journal of Nutrition* 108, no. 4, pp. 692–98. doi:10.1017/s0007114512001808

Tsukaguchi, H., T. Tokui, B. Mackenzie, U.V. Berger, X.Z. Chen, Y. Wang, R.F. Brubaker, and M.A. Hediger. 1999. "A family of Mammalian Na+-Dependent L-Ascorbic Acid Transporters." *Nature* 399, no. 6731, pp. 70–5. doi:10.1038/19986

Valkonen, M.M., and T. Kuusi. 2000. "Vitamin C Prevents the Acute Atherogenic Effects of Passive Smoking." *Free Radical Biology and Medicine* 28, no. 3, pp. 428–36. doi:10.1016/s0891-5849(99)00260-9

Van Lente, F. 2000. "Markers of Inflammation as Predictors in Cardiovascular Disease." *Clinica Chimica Acta* 293, no. 1–2, pp. 31–52. doi:10.1016/s0009-8981(99)00236-3

Van Schoor, N.M., and P. Lips. 2011. "Worldwide Vitamin D Status." *Best Practice & Research Clinical Endocrinology & Metabolism* 25, no. 4, pp. 671–80. doi:10.1016/j.beem.2011.06.007

Wallace, T.C., and D. MacKay. 2013. "Dietary Supplement Regulation in the United States." In *SpringerBriefs in Food, Health, and Nutrition*, eds. T.C. MacKay, D. Al-Mondhiry, R. Nguyen, H. Griffiths, and J.C. Wallace, 1–38. Cham: Springer International Publishing.

Warensjo, E., L. Byberg, H. Melhus, R. Gedeborg, H. Mallmin, A. Wolk, and K. Michaelsson. 2011. "Dietary Calcium Intake and Risk of Fracture and Osteoporosis: Prospective Longitudinal Cohort Study." *BMJ* 342, pp. d1473. doi:10.1136/bmj.d1473

Welten, D.C., H.C. Kemper, G.B. Post, and W.A. van Staveren. 1995. "A Meta-Analysis of the Effect of Calcium Intake on Bone Mass in Young and Middle Aged Females and Males." *Nutrition Journal* 125, no. 11, pp. 2802–13. doi:10.1007/BF02499982

Wood, A.D., K.R. Secombes, F. Thies, L. Aucott, A.J. Black, A. Mavroeidi, W.G. Simpson, W.D. Fraser, D.M. Reid, and H.M. Macdonald. 2012. "Vitamin D3 Supplementation Has No Effect on Conventional Cardiovascular Risk Factors: A Parallel-Group, Double-Blind, Placebo-Controlled RCT." *Journal of Clinical Endocrinology & Metabolism* 97, no. 10, pp. 3557–68. doi:10.1210/jc.2012-2126

World Health Organization. 2012. *World Health Statistics 2012.* The World Health Statistics Series, Geneva, Switzerland: World Health Organization.

Wu-Wong, J.R., M. Nakane, J. Ma, X. Ruan, and P.E. Kroeger. 2006. "Effects of Vitamin D Analogs on Gene Expression Profiling in Human Coronary Artery Smooth Muscle Cells." *Atherosclerosis* 186, no. 1, pp. 20–8. doi:10.1016/j.atherosclerosis.2005.06.046

Zittermann, A., S.S. Schleithoff, G. Tenderich, H.K. Berthold, R. Körfer, and P. Stehle. 2003. "Low Vitamin D Status: A Contributing Factor in the Pathogenesis of Congestive Heart Failure?" *Journal of the American College of Cardiology* 41, no. 1, pp. 105–12.

CHAPTER 3

Survey of the 20 Most Common Dietary Supplements—Specialty Supplements

Overview

This chapter reviews the varied classes and properties of specialty supplements. Specialty supplements are dietary supplement ingredients that do not neatly fit into other supplement categories. In this chapter, we review omega-3 fatty acids, fiber, probiotics, glucosamine, and chondroitin, and coenzyme Q10. The background, properties, and clinical trials involving each ingredient are discussed. The safety of each are also reviewed.

Introduction

Supplements that do not neatly fit into other supplement categories are called specialty supplements in the industry. Included in the list of the 20 most popular supplements are five supplements that fall into this category: omega-3 oils, fiber, probiotics, glucosamine and chondroitin, and coenzyme Q10. In this chapter we review these five supplements and include a discussion of their function in the body, the reasons people use them and if these reasons are supported by clinical studies, and their safety. You may notice that, in this chapter, an emphasis is placed on discussing the evidence behind the use of omega-3 oils as dietary supplements. This is done because of the controversy over some of the health claims associated with these products. As with most dietary supplements, there is evidence for and against the claims made about them. We will try to present an objective look at the evidence on either side. Keep in mind that our discussion of any of the following supplements is not exhaustive, and there is a lot more to say and more research to review than can be included in this book. Nevertheless, it is hoped that just enough information is presented to spark even more interest into the fascinating research behind specialty supplements.

Omega-3 Fatty Acids

Background

Essential fatty acids (EFAs) are a group of nutritionally essential polyunsaturated fatty acids required for proper growth, maintenance, and function of the body. EFAs include both omega-3 and omega-6 fatty acids. The terms omega-3 and omega-6 designate their structures and refer to the position of the double bond relative to the terminal, or "omega," carbon.

Omega-3s and omega-6s are precursors to a group of hormone-like lipid compounds called eicosanoids; these include prostaglandins, thromboxanes, and leukotrienes. Eicosanoids play critical roles in regulating many complex physiological processes such as immunity and inflammation, algesia, cell division and growth, blood clotting, labor and delivery, secretion of digestive juices and hormones, and movement of substances like calcium into and out of cells.

As omega-3 fatty acid supplements are the focus of this chapter, we will forego discussion of omega-6 fatty acids, which are rarely consumed as a dietary supplement. Dietary sources of omega-3 fatty acids include flax seeds, walnuts, and fatty fish. Omega-3s from plant sources is in the form of alpha-linolenic acid (ALA). Fatty fish provide eicosapentaenoic acid (EPA) and docosahexaenoic acid (DHA). The fatty acids EPA and DHA are by far the most commonly supplemented omega-3s.

Fish oil is the most plentiful source of EPA and DHA, and the majority of omega-3 products are sourced from various abundant species of fish, sardines and anchovies being the most common. Fish oil supplements often contain small amounts of vitamin E to improve stability and shelf life. Some omega-3 products do not contain oil from fish but are sourced from other marine animals including krill and marine algae. The source and processing of the oils can lead to different forms of fatty acids in the finished product. For example, the majority of fish oil supplements provide EPA and DHA in the form of triglycerides. Krill and some algae on the other hand provide EPA and DHA in the form of phospholipids. This difference impacts both digestibility and absorption.

Fish oil and oil derived from krill and some algae involve different digestion processes according to the differences in their chemical form. The digestive lipolytic enzymes pancreatic phospholipase A2 and lipase are involved in the digestion of phospholipids and triglycerides respectively. These two enzymes differ both in nature and activity.

Each enzyme reacts in very specific ways with its substrate. Fish oils are somewhat resistant, at least in vitro, to digestion by lipases because their structure partly obstructs the site where the enzyme acts on them (Bottino 1957), whereas phospholipase A2, which is required to digest phospholipids, is not influenced by the structure of the fatty acids because it acts at a different site that is not obstructed. This facilitates the digestion of phospholipids compared to that of triglycerides.

Phospholipids also affect the oil's solubility. Krill oil, for example, is naturally emulsified by its phospholipid content. Emulsification improves digestion and absorption of EPA and DHA because of the increased solubility of the krill fatty acids compared to fatty acids in triglyceride form (Garaiova et al. 2007; Schuchardt et al. 2011). The emulsified and more water soluble state of krill oil increases its exposure to digestive enzymes and thus diminishes gastric clearance time (Raatz et al. 2009). This can also have a significant impact on "fishy burp back" that some fish oil users experience, which causes many to stop taking it. The increased solubility of phospholipid oils allows it to mix with stomach contents leaving less to float at the top as a layer of oil thus reducing fishy burp back and improving compliance.

Rationale for Supplementation

Achieving Nutritionally Adequate Levels of EPA and DHA

EFA deficiency manifests in a variety of bodily systems and tissues. Symptoms include scaly skin rashes, alopecia, brittle nails, infertility, neurological dysfunction, altered immunity, and decreased growth in children and infants (Smit, Muskiet, and Rudy Boersma 2004). Though outright deficiency is not common in developed countries, an inadequate intake is common and can contribute to a number of chronic health problems. It has been estimated that as many as 96,000 deaths per year in the United States can be attributed to inadequate intake of EPA and DHA (Danaei et al. 2009). Epidemiological data suggests that the average American consumes less than 100 mg/day of EPA and DHA (USDA 2012). This level is well below the published recommendations of 250 to 500 mg/day of combined EPA and DHA (USDA 2010).

Some suggest increasing plant based sources of omega-3s, which provide ALA, will provide adequate EPA and DHA. This strategy however is often ineffective. Technically speaking, EPA is a nonessential n-3 fatty acid as long as ALA is consumed in the diet. In humans however, there is tremendous interindividual variability in the ability to enzymatically convert ALA into EPA and DHA (see Figure 3.1). Research indicates that conversion of ALA to EPA and DHA may be as low as 0.3 and 0.01 percent respectively (Hussein 2005). These conversion rates generally do

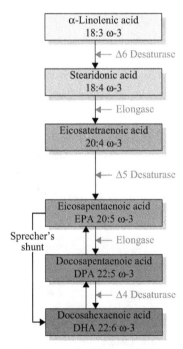

Figure 3.1 Enzymatic conversion of ALA into EPA and DHA

not provide optimal levels of EPA and DHA, thus putting these fatty acids in the category of conditionally essential nutrients. Adequate intake of EPA and DHA can be accomplished by consuming fatty fish at least twice weekly and taking marine sourced omega-3 dietary supplements.

Improving the Ratio of Omega-6 and Omega-3 Fatty Acids in the Diet

Both omega-3 and omega-6 fatty acids are precursors to eicosanoids; however, those derived from omega-3s and omega-6s lead to different subgroups of eicosanoids with sometimes opposing physiological effects. Generally speaking, eicosanoids derived from omega-6 fatty acids are proinflammatory, while eicosanoids derived from omega-3 fatty acids are anti-inflammatory (see Figure 3.2). It is believed that the ratio of omega-3 derived eicosanoids and omega-6 derived eicosanoids can impact systemic levels of inflammation (Patterson et al. 2012).

An increase in the consumption of processed foods and omega-6 rich vegetable oils over the last few decades has increased the omega-6 to omega-3 ratio (~15:1) in the American diet as well as many other developed countries (Blasbalg et al. 2011). The optimum ratio is believed

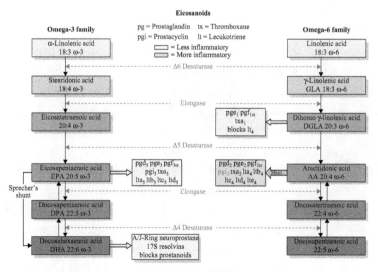

Figure 3.2 Metabolic pathway of omega-3 and omega-6 fatty acids showing pro- and anti-inflammatory eicosanoids

to be closer to 1.4:1 (Molendi-Coste, Legry, and Leclercq 2011). Increases in the prevalence of chronic inflammatory diseases such as rheumatoid arthritis (RA), obesity, nonalcoholic fatty liver disease, cardiovascular disease, inflammatory bowel disease (IBS), and Alzheimer's disease has coincided with this perturbation of the omega-6 to omega-3 ratio in Western diets (Patterson et al. 2012). Without a drastic change in dietary habits, omega-3 supplementation is required to bring the omega-6 to omega-3 ratio back down to a level that may reduce the incidence and prevalence of chronic inflammatory diseases.

Finally, there is evidence that postpartum depression (PPD) may be associated with the dietary ratio of omega-6 and omega-3s. PPD is a serious condition affecting the emotional state and maternal behaviors of the mother. PPD can increase the risk of psychopathologies and developmental problems in the child. Some research has shown that the prevalence of PPD more than doubles in women with a dietary omega-6 to omega-3 ratio greater than 9:1 (da Rocha and Gilberto 2012).

Achieving Tissue Levels of EPA and DHA Associated with Reduced Cardiovascular Risk

Perhaps the strongest evidence for the value of supplementation with omega-3s is for cardiovascular health. Mechanistically, it has been demonstrated that EPA and DHA could contribute to preventing cardiovascular disease through several mechanisms. DiNicolantonio and colleagues have provided a list of many mechanisms by which EPA and DHA could be affecting cardiovascular health (see Table 3.1) (DiNicolantonio et al. 2014).

The aforementioned mechanisms by which EP and DHA may reduce cardiovascular risk are associated with and dependent upon the amount of EPA and DHA in tissues and cells. It is thought (and data supports) the notion that a certain level of EPA and DHA in tissues and cells is required before protective effects are seen (Harris and von Schacky 2004). The level of EPA and DHA in tissues and cells can be expressed as a percentage derived by use of the Omega-3 Index (O3I). The O3I is a measure of the combined percentage of EPA and DHA in the total fatty acids in

Table 3.1 Possible mechanisms by which dietary EPA and DHA may improve cardiovascular health

How dietary EPA and DHA may improve cardiovascular health:
Reduction of plasma and postprandial triglycerides
Lowered heart rate and systolic and diastolic blood pressure
Reduced risk of heart failure
Improved left ventricular diastolic filling
Improved left ventricular ejection fraction
Improved left ventricular end-systolic volume
Improved peak oxygen consumption
Improved myocardial efficiency
Lowered myocardial oxygen demand
Improved hepatic steatosis and improved insulin resistance
Lowered systemic vascular resistance, improved arterial compliance, and improved endothelial function
Reduced inflammatory cytokines (e.g., serum amyloid A [SAA], SAA low-density lipoprotein cholesterol, C-reactive protein [CRP], and interleukin-6)
Resolution of inflammation through increased production of resolvins, protectins, docosatrienes, and neuroprotectins
Decreased arachidonic acid (AA)-derived eicosanoids such as thromboxanes, 2-series prostaglandins, and 4-series leukotrienes
Reduced intracranial stenosis
Reduced ventricular arrhythmias
Atrial fibrillation
Antiatherogenic effects
Antithrombotic effects

red blood cell membranes. The O3I is directly related to dietary intake of EPA and DHA (Flock et al. 2013). Data presented in Table 3.2 suggests that a desirable target value for the O3I is ≥8 percent and an undesirable level of ≤4 percent (see Table 3.2) (Harris 2015).

The data from Table 3.2 illustrates the importance of adequate omega-3 fatty acids in the diet. As of this writing, the O3I has not been officially recognized by the American Heart Association or other author-itative bodies, such as the American Medical Association, as an official predictor of cardiovascular risk. It is very likely this will change in the near future in the light of currently available and newly published evidence of its predictive value.

Table 3.2 The association of red blood cell omega-3 fatty acids (O3I)
and cardiovascular risk

Higher O3I:
Is inversely associated with triglyceride levels
Is inversely associated with heart rate
Is inversely associated with blood pressure
Is inversely associated with levels of inflammatory markers
Is inversely associated with risk of death from cardiovascular disease in interventional and epidemiological studies
Is inversely associated with risk of total mortality in coronary heart disease (CHD) patients
Is inversely associated with sudden cardiac death
Is inversely associated with reduced 17-year risk for sudden cardiac death independent of other CHD risk factors and showed greater predictive value than total cholesterol, LDL-C, HDL-C, triglycerides, homocysteine, and CRP
Is inversely associated with risk of in-hospital ventricular fibrillation and sudden cardiac arrest in postmyocardial infarction (MI) patients
Is typical of Japan, a country with the world's greatest longevity (4 years > U.S.) and very low CHD death rates. (O3I average 9 to 10 percent)

Pro-Resolving Lipid Mediators

Pro-resolving lipid mediators are molecules enzymatically derived from
EPA, DHA, and the omega-6 fatty acid AA. Increasing the intake of EPA
and DHA may lead to active resolution of inflammation by way of pro-
resolving lipid mediators (Mas et al. 2012). I will generalize the various
pro-resolving lipid mediators derived from EPA, DHA, and AA simply
as "resolvins" for the sake of simplicity; nevertheless, it should be noted
that there are at least four recognized classes of these lipid mediators,
namely lipoxins from AA, resolvins and protectins from EPA and DHA,
and maresins, a novel pro-resolving mediator derived from DHA that is
released from macrophages.

It was believed until recently that the resolution of inflammation was
a passive process. It was thought that the dissipation of inflammatory
cytokines would eventually decrease the inflammatory activity until it had
resolved, much like a fire is left to "burn itself out." More recently it has
come to light that the resolution of inflammation is an active process

involving locally produced bioactive compounds that actively resolve inflammation, much like a fire extinguisher quenches a fire (Serhan et al. 2014). EPA and DHA are the precursors to these resolvins. It may be that the levels of resolvins are dependent on the tissue levels of its precursors EPA and DHA, which are known to be influenced by dietary intake. This topic is the focus of recent research and initial results indicate that supplementation with EPA and DHA is a viable approach to increasing resolvin levels (Mas et al. 2012). Currently, much is being learned about these and other pro-resolving mediators. For the time being however, for those that wish to act proactively to support healthy and appropriate inflammatory activity supplementing with EPA and DHA is a logical option.

Other Potential Health Benefits of Supplementing with Omega-3 Fatty Acids

Mood and Cognitive Function.   Evidence from animal and human studies show that omega-3 deficiency leads to impaired neuronal function of serotoninergic and dopaminergic pathways in the brain (Patrick and Ames 2015). In addition, several epidemiological studies have demonstrated an inverse relationship between fatty fish consumption and depressive disorders. Over a decade ago an inverse association between fish consumption and prevalence of major depression across nine countries was reported (Hibbeln 1998). Since then, several epidemiological studies on oily fish consumption and depression demonstrated a significant inverse correlation between oily fish consumption and prevalence and incidence of depression and bipolar disorder, setting a threshold of vulnerability of about 650 mg/day. Meta-analyses have concluded that n-3 PUFA supplements may be beneficial in treating unipolar and bipolar depressive disorders (Lin 2007). At least one meta-analysis however did not come to the same conclusion (Appleton et al. 2006).

There has been considerable interest in the effects of omega-3 supplementation on attention deficit hyperactivity disorder (ADHD) in children. ADHD is estimated to effect as many as 10 percent of school age children. Accumulating evidence from epidemiological, biochemical, and intervention studies suggests that a diet inadequate in the omega-3 fatty acids EPA and DHA may have a detrimental effect on children's behavior and cognitive development (Schuchardt et al. 2010) (Ryan et al. 2010). Data is also available showing reduced levels of EPA and DHA in children exhibiting ADHD. Randomized controlled trials and meta-analysis, however, have shown mixed results: some show significant improvements in cognitive performance and behavior, while others fail to show meaningful benefits (Bloch and Ahmad 2011; Gillies et al. 2012).

Eye Health.   There is some evidence that people who consume fish oil from dietary fish at least twice a week have a reduced risk of developing age-related macular degeneration (AMD). Most epidemiological studies show an inverse relationship between dietary intake of EPA and DHA and prevalence of AMD. Both an increase in dietary intake and frequency of dietary intake resulted in a lowered risk of AMD progression (Liu et al. 2011).

Asthma.   Inflammatory eicosanoids derived from omega-6 fatty acids are believed to play a role in the pathology of asthma. Supplementation with omega-3 fatty acids can reduce the production of inflammatory eicosanoids and, in turn, reduce the inflammatory potential of tissues. Clinical trials have been conducted to explore the benefits of omega-3 supplementation on the etiology of asthma. A meta-analysis and systematic review failed to show consistent benefit in subjects with asthma following fish oil supplementation (Thien, Woods, and Abramson 2002). Some clinical trials however, show that taking fish oil supplements improves peak flow and reduces medication use and cough in children with asthma (Broughton et al. 1997).

Rheumatoid Arthritis.   RA is a disease characterized by significant inflammation of the joints. The ability of omega-3 fatty acids to reduce inflammatory eicosanoids makes it a logical candidate for reducing the symptoms of RA. Many studies on the effects of omega-3 fatty acids as an adjunct treatment for RA have been conducted, including a trial using krill oil. According to one placebo-controlled trial, krill oil significantly improved measures of pain, stiffness, joint function as assessed by the Western Ontario and McMaster Universities Osteoarthritis Index (WOMAC). Krill oil also reduced the use of rescue medicines and reduced the systemic inflammatory marker CRP levels compared to placebo (Deutsch 2007). Reviews of these RA intervention trials have concluded that there is some benefit derived from supplementing with omega-3s, characterized by a reduction in pain, stiffness, and pain upon examination (Fortin et al. 1995). Two meta-analysis of RA clinical trials agree with the aforementioned reviews. In these analyses, supplementation significantly decreased the number of painful and tender joints on physical examination (Fortin et al. 1995; Goldberg and Katz 2007). Taken together, there is good evidence that supplementation with omega-3s improves symptoms of RA.

Pregnancy. In a review of fifteen randomized controlled trials with over 8,454 pregnant women, supplementation with omega-3 long-chain polyunsaturated fatty acids was associated with 26 percent lower risk of early preterm birth and moderately increased birth weight compared with placebo (Imhoff-Kunsch et al. 2012).

Omega-3 supplementation during pregnancy substantially increases fetal DHA concentration at birth. Two randomized controlled trials have shown that DHA supplementation during pregnancy also significantly improves infant neurocognitive development. One striking study was able to show that supplementation with omega-3s during pregnancy and lactation increases a child's IQ at 4 years of age (Helland et al. 2003). It should be mentioned however that when the children are left to consume a typical diet without omega-3 supplementation, the differences in IQ disappear by age seven (Helland et al. 2008).

The previous list is only a small sample of conditions that have been investigated for beneficial effects of omega-3 fatty acids. To examine them all is beyond the scope of this work. The preceding does however represent the more common potential health benefits for which people chose to supplement with omega-3 fatty acids.

Safety

Because most omega-3 supplements are taken in the form of fish oil, the potential for these products to contain ocean contaminants such as methylmercury, Polychlorinated biphenyls (PCBs), and dioxins has been noted. Several independent laboratory analyses in the United States have found most commercially available omega-3 supplements to be free of methylmercury, PCBs, and dioxins (Melanson et al. 2005). The absence of methylmercury in fish oil supplements can be explained by the fact that mercury accumulates in the muscle rather than the fat of the fish. It should be noted that fish body oils contain lower levels of PCBs and other fat-soluble contaminants than fish liver oils. Additionally, fish oils that have been more highly refined and deodorized by a process called molecular distillation also contain very low levels of PCBs.

An evidence report or technology assessment conducted by Tufts University reviewed 148 studies to evaluate adverse events not including fishy aftertaste-from the use of omega-3 fatty acid supplements (typically fish oils) (Wang and Chung 2004). The report included about 10,000 subjects who had taken omega-3 supplements in various forms and dosages ranging from 0.3 to 8 g/day for at least 1 week to more than 7 years. Half of all studies reviewed reported no adverse events. Less than 7 percent of subjects reported side effects, and those that were reported were minor, mainly gastrointestinal in nature (such as diarrhea) and were associated with higher doses of oil. Although bleeding is a theoretical concern, this was not borne out by the evidence. All adverse events related to consumption of fish-oil or ALA supplements consist mainly of stomach upset and can be managed by reducing the dose or discontinuing the supplement.

Fiber

Background

Fiber is generally considered to include all nondigestible vegetable matter in the diet. This includes polysaccharides, lignin, oligosaccharides, and

SPECIALTY SUPPLEMENTS   77

Table 3.3 Examples of foods containing soluble and insoluble fiber

Soluble	Insoluble
Apples	Fruit skins
Ripe Bananas	Unripe Bananas
Pears	Potato skins
Citrus fruits	Brussels sprouts
Berries	Carrots
Cherries	Celery
Dates	Spinach
Figs	Sweet potato
Prunes	Cabbage
Onions	Cauliflower
Sweet potatoes	Nuts and Seeds
Potatoes	Wheat bran
Carrots	Corn bran
Nuts	Legumes (beans)
Oat meal	Rye
Legumes (beans)	Whole-grains

resistant starches (Jones, Lineback, and Levine 2006). Fiber is made up of components of plant cell walls. Fresh fruits, vegetables, whole grains, nuts, and legumes are our primary source of dietary fiber. Fibers are classified as water soluble and water insoluble. Most fibrous foods are not exclusively soluble or insoluble. Soluble fiber, such as fruit pectin, can be fermented in the colon, and insoluble fibers, such as wheat bran, may only be fermented to a limited extent. Fermentation is the process of being broken down or metabolized by glut flora. Soluble fiber that specifically enhances the growth of beneficial bacteria in the digestive tract is known as prebiotic fiber. Prebiotic fibers include the oligosaccharides and resistant starches such as inulin and high-amylose maize, respectively. A short list of food sources of dietary fiber appears in Table 3.3.

Fiber supplements contain fiber isolated and extracted from foods and vegetable matter. Generally they are in the form of powders that can be added to liquids and drunk. Unlike foods, fiber supplements generally do not have both soluble and insoluble characteristics. This stems from the fact that they are isolated substances rather than a mix of different food stuffs. Fiber supplements can be classified according to their characteristics:

Soluble Fiber Supplements:

Fiber supplements, as described by McRorie, can be categorized into three classes based on the following characteristics: solubility, degree and rate of fermentation, viscosity, and gel formation (McRorie 2015a, 2015b).

Viscous or gel-forming, readily fermented fiber: These fibers dissolve in water and form a viscous gel. They increase viscosity of stomach contents to slow nutrient absorption and through this means may improve glycemic control. These fibers may also lower elevated serum cholesterol when combined with a low fat low cholesterol diet. They are readily fermented, which increases short chain fatty acid production as well as gas. Fermentation results in loss of gel and waterholding capacity, and thus, they have no significant laxative effect or retained gel to attenuate diarrhea. Examples include A-glucans from oatmeal and barley, and raw guar gum.

Viscous or gel-forming, nonfermented fiber: These fibers readily dissolve in water and form a viscous gel. They increase viscosity of stomach contents to slow nutrient absorption and through this means may improve glycemic control. These fibers may also lower elevated serum cholesterol when combined with a low fat low cholesterol diet. These fibers are not fermented by gut bacteria; therefore, they do not cause gas production or short chain fatty acid production. Because this type of fiber is not fermented, it remains gelled throughout the large intestine providing the unique benefit of reducing both constipation and diarrhea. An example is psyllium from psyllium husk.

Nonviscous, readily fermented: These fibers dissolve in water but do not increase viscosity of stomach contents; so they do not provide any gel-dependent benefits such as slowed nutrient absorption. They are rapidly and completely fermented in the small and large intestines. Once fermented, the fiber is no longer present in the stool. They can cause rapid gas formation and increased flatulence in large doses. Short chain fatty acid production is increased, and perhaps most importantly, the numbers of beneficial bacteria in the gut is also increased. They produce no laxative effect at normal doses and have no short-term benefits for constipation or diarrhea.

Examples include the prebiotic fibers such as inulin, short chain fructo-oligosaccharides (SCFOS), and resistant starches.

Insoluble Fiber:

Insoluble fiber has fewer variable characteristics. There is essentially only one class of insoluble fiber:

Insoluble, poorly fermented: These fibers do not dissolve in water (no water-holding capacity). They are poorly fermented and thus have little impact on gut flora. They can exert a laxative effect by mechanical irritation or stimulation of gut mucosa if particles are sufficiently large and coarse. Small smooth fiber particles (e.g., wheat bran flour or bread) have no significant laxative effect. Insoluble fiber does not gel or alter viscosity and thus does not provide other (gel-dependent) fiber health benefits such as reduced cholesterol and glycemic control. Examples include wheat bran, skins of fruits and tubers, and leafy green vegetables.

Rationale for Supplementation

Large Bowel Function

Constipation and diarrhea are two common large bowel dysfunctions that can be improved with fiber supplementation. The functional benefits of fiber, with the exception of prebiotics, are due to the fiber's physical effects in the small and large intestine. Insoluble fibers such as wheat bran exert a laxative effect by increasing stool weight and mechanical irritation or stimulation of gut mucosa if particles are sufficiently large and coarse. Decreased transit time through the digestive tract and particularly the large bowel may decrease the incidence of large bowel disorders such as constipation, diverticulitis, and large bowel cancers. Fibers such as psyllium are gel forming and can "normalize" stool by absorbing excess water in the large bowel, reducing the frequency of bowel movements.

The majority of clinical benefits provided by dietary fiber, whether it is from whole foods or supplements, are due to the viscous properties of select fibers. The viscosity of certain fibers slows the digestion of foods by preventing bulk absorption of nutrients across the intestinal lumen.

This can have a significant effect on glycemic control as well as cholesterol levels. Both of these are related to one's risk of cardiovascular disease.

Glycemic Control

Glucose obtained from the carbohydrates in a meal is normally rapidly absorbed in the most proximal end of the small intestine. This rapid absorption results in a correspondingly rapid rise in blood glucose levels. Even in healthy individuals, this rapid rise in blood glucose levels produces a spike in insulin levels. High insulin causes a rapid decline in blood glucose that transiently falls below baseline levels, causing temporary hypoglycemia. Viscous gel-forming fiber can dramatically reduce this rollercoaster in blood glucose levels. By forming a gel, glucose is trapped within the viscous bolus and absorption is dramatically slowed. With the addition of a gel-forming fiber, absorption of glucose takes place along the entire length of the small intestine, reducing peak glucose and insulin levels and suppressing appetite.

Regular intake of a viscous gel-forming fiber supplement can also have significant benefits for long-term management of blood sugar levels. An eight-week, placebo-controlled clinical study evaluated psyllium for improved blood sugar control in 49 patients already being treated for type 2 diabetes (Ziai et al. 2005). After 8 weeks of taking 5 g of psyllium twice a day, fasting blood glucose was significantly decreased compared to the placebo group. Hemoglobin A1c and measure of long-term blood glucose levels also showed a significant decrease versus placebo. Interestingly, the improvements seen with psyllium supplementation were additive to the effects of the oral medications these subjects were already taking to control blood sugar levels.

Cholesterol

It has been demonstrated that a 1 percent reduction in serum levels of LDL-cholesterol corresponds to a 1 to 2 percent reduction in occurrence of CHD events, making LDL-cholesterol a good biomarker for assessment of CHD risk (Kendall, Esfahani, and Jenkins 2010). Supplementing with fiber can have a significant effect on cholesterol levels.

Viscous gel-forming fibers have significant hypocholesterolemic effects, whereas nonviscous fibers do not. Two gel-forming fibers, Guar gum and psyllium, have been heavily studied for their effects on cholesterol. Anderson et al. have provided information on the net impact of soluble viscous fibers on cholesterol (change with fiber treatment minus change with placebo treatment) (Anderson et al. 2009). A review of over 40 clinical trials on guar gum indicated that intakes ranging from 9 to 30 g/day, divided into at least three servings per day, were associated with a weighted mean reduction of 10.6 percent for LDL-cholesterol values. For pectin, consumption of 12 to 24 g/day in divided doses was associated with a 13 percent reduction in LDL-cholesterol. Barley beta-glucan intake of 5 g/day in divided doses was associated with an 11.1 percent reduction in LDL-cholesterol values. Although less data is available for hydroxypropyl methylcellulose, trials indicate that 5 g/day in divided doses decreases LDL-cholesterol values by 8.5 percent.

Microbiome

Some fibers are able to selectively increase the populations of good bacteria in the digestive tract. We call these fibers prebiotics. Prebiotics are not classified in the same manner as "bulk" fibers. Prebiotics are classified simply by their ability to selectively increase good microflora. The current official definition of a prebiotic is "A dietary prebiotic is a selectively fermented ingredient that results in specific changes in the composition and activity of the GI microbiota thus conferring benefit(s) upon host health" (Gibson et al. 2010).

The concept of prebiotics is rather new in terms of the history of discoveries about human health (Gibson and Roberfroid 1995). Nevertheless, the number of studies published on prebiotics has increased from one in 1995 to over 340 in 2014. The growth in our understanding has increased dramatically just in the last 10 years; for example, the number of published studies has increased by a factor of six since 2005. Out of this research has come a range of potential health areas that are or may be impacted by the use of prebiotics. Table 3.4 lists some of these health areas being studied with prebiotics (Roberfroid et al. 2010).

Table 3.4 The primary health areas and conditions as targets for prebiotic benefits

Improvement and stabilization of gut microbiota composition
Improvement of intestinal functions (stool bulking, stool regularity, stool consistency)
Increase in mineral absorption and improvement of bone health (bone mineral density)
Modulation of gastrointestinal peptides production, energy metabolism, and satiety
Initiation (after birth) and regulation and modulation of immune functions
Improvement of intestinal barrier functions, reduction of metabolic endotoxemia
Reduction of risk of intestinal infections
Reduction of risk of obesity, type 2 diabetes, metabolic syndrome, and so on
Reduction of risk of and improvement in the management of intestinal inflammation
Reduction of risk of colon cancer

Safety

Because fiber is a natural component of foods that we consume every day, there has never really been any suspicion that it might be unsafe. Rather, fibers are evaluated in terms of "intestinal acceptability" (Coussement 1999). Intestinal acceptability of fiber is determined mainly by two criteria: (1) The osmotic effect, which leads to an increased draw of water into the colon. Smaller molecules exert a higher osmotic pressure and bring more water into the colon. (2) The fermentability of the fiber, which leads to the buildup of fermentation products, mainly short-chain fatty acids and gases. Slowly fermenting compounds appear to be easier to tolerate than their fast fermenting analogs. This would explain why inulin is easier to tolerate than oligofructose.

The intake of fermentable fibers is self-limiting because of flatulence or gas. For nonfermentable fibers it is loose stools or diarrhea. Dietary fibers are considered nontoxic and are considered safe in food as dietary supplements. Synthetic fibers, although less common, must demonstrate their safety by applying for generally recognized as safe (GRAS) status with the Food and Drug Administration (FDA). GRAS is the label given to food components and ingredients approved for human consumption by the FDA. A synthetic or semisynthetic fiber intended to be used as a dietary supplement would also have to apply for and receive approval as a "new dietary ingredient" (NDI) from the FDA.

Probiotics

Background

Bacterial colonization of the gut and skin begins at birth and continues throughout life with notable age-specific changes. Bacteria are normal inhabitants of the gastrointestinal tract, where more than 1,000 bacterial species are found. These resident intestinal microflora do not normally have any acute adverse effects, and some of them have been shown to be necessary for maintaining the health and well-being of their host.

The notion of the importance of probiotics is certainly not new. By 1886, Escherich had described the microbiota and early colonization of the infant gastrointestinal tract and suggested their benefit for digestion, whereas Döderlein was probably the first scientist to suggest the beneficial association of vaginal bacteria by production of lactic acid from sugars, thereby preventing or inhibiting the growth of pathogenic bacteria (Goktepe, Juneja, and Ahmedna 2006).

The idea that certain bacteria could be supplemented orally to improve intestinal health was first proposed in 1907 by Eli Metchnikoff, a Russian born Nobel Prize recipient working at the Pasteur Institute (FAO/WHO 2001; Metchnikoff 1907). He observed, "The dependence of the intestinal microbes on the food makes it possible to adopt measures to modify the flora in our bodies and to replace the harmful microbes by useful microbes" (Metchnikoff 1907). In spite of this early understanding of the potential benefits of ingesting beneficial bacteria, the term "probiotic" meaning "for life" was not coined until the mid-1960s, (Lilly and Stillwell 1965). In the intervening century since Metchnikoff's insightful proposals and more particularly the last two decades, research on probiotics has progressed considerably and significant advances have been made in the identification and characterization of specific probiotic strains and substantiation of health claims relating to their consumption.

A commonly accepted definition of a probiotic is "Live microorganisms which when administered in adequate amounts confer a health benefit on the host" (FAO/WHO 2001). Only a relatively small number of bacterial species meet this definition. Probiotics are primarily bacteria from the lactobacillus, bifidobacterium, and bacillus genera. However,

Lactococcus, Streptococcus, and *Enterococcus* species, as well as some non-pathogenic strains of *Escherichia coli* and certain yeast strains, may also act as probiotics. A brief list of examples of bacterial probiotics with origins is presented in Table 3.5.

Table 3.5 Bacterial probiotics currently sold as supplements (not exhaustive)

Species strain	Origin
Lactobacillus acidophilus DDS-1 strain	Human
Lactobacillus brevis	Unknown
L. brevis is mainly found in food. Environmentally, it can be found on dairy farms in raw milk, especially in bovine feces; however it rarely teams up with eukaryotes in a symbiotic way. Mostly it is found in proximity with other lactic acid bacteria, in a variety of foods	
Lactobacillus bulgaricus	Dairy
Lactobacillus casei	Unknown
L. casei can be found in various environments such as raw and fermented dairy products, intestinal tracts and reproductive systems of humans and animals, and fresh and fermented plant products	
Lactobacillus helveticus	Dairy
Lactobacillus plantarum	Plant
Lactobacillus paracasei	Unknown
L. paracasei can be found in dairy products, sewage, silage, and humans.	
Lactobacillus rhamnosus	Human
Lactobacillus salivarius	Human
Bacillus coagulans (formerly "*Lactobacillus sporogenes*")	Soil
Bacillus subtilis soil (formerly *Vibrio subtilis*)	Soil
Bifidobacterium bifidum (formerly *Lactobacillus bifidus*)	Dairy
Bifidobacterium breve (*B. Breve* was originally isolated from healthy human infant intestine)	Unknown
Bifidobacterium lactis (infantis)	Human
Bifidobacterium longum	Human
Lactococcus lactis	Unknown
L. lactis (formerly *S. faecium*) is a spherical-shaped, Gram-positive bacterium used widely for industrial production of fermented dairy products such as milk, cheese, and yogurt. It can also be found in the wild on plants and within the digestive tract of cows. It is believed that in nature, *L. lactis* stays dormant on plant surfaces awaiting to be ingested along with the plant into the animal's gastrointestinal tract, where it becomes active and multiplies intensively	

Enterococcus faecium	Unknown
E. faecium is a species of gram-positive, coccoid bacteria whose organisms are normal flora of the human intestinal tract	
Streptococcus thermophilus	Dairy
Pediococcus acidilacti	Unknown
Found in plant and milk products	

Not all bacteria qualify as probiotics, even if they are not harmful when ingested. To qualify as a probiotic an organism should show some combination of the following characteristics (Dash 2009):

- Be resistant to gastric acidity
- Be resistant to bile acid
- Demonstrate bile salt hydrolase activity
- Adhere to mucus and human epithelial lining of the gut
- Possess antimicrobial activity against potentially pathogenic bacteria
- Possess the ability to reduce pathogen adhesion to surfaces in the gastrointestinal tract
- Demonstrate beneficial immune modulating ability.

This list of potential characteristics in not comprehensive. For example, the gut brain axis is now being intensely studied as is the impact of gut bacteria on metabolism and obesity. As our understanding of the microbiome grows, it may soon be that due to complexity, no single list of characteristics will be adequate as inclusion criteria for *all* potential probiotics.

Rationale for Supplementation

Major probiotic mechanisms of action include fermentation of dietary fiber, enhancement of the epithelial barrier, increased adhesion to intestinal mucosa, concomitant inhibition of pathogen adhesion, competitive exclusion of pathogenic microorganisms, production of antimicrobial substances, and modulation of the immune system (Backhed et al. 2005; Bermudez-Brito et al. 2012).

Fermentation of Dietary Fiber

The cell walls of plant material that we eat contain complex carbohydrate molecules that we cannot digest; we call these carbohydrates dietary fiber. Our ability to digest complex carbohydrates is dependent on the type of enzymes that we produce. We do not produce all the enzymes necessary to break down all the different types of carbohydrates that we eat. Probiotics along with the endogenous bacteria in the digestive tract do however produce numerous enzymes that are able to break down simple as well as very complex carbohydrates in a process called fermentation. Without this help from our gut bacteria, all dietary fiber we eat would pass through the digestive tract much like insoluble fiber. This would dramatically increase the laxative effects of eating nonanimal foods. Probiotics, by their own action and by enhancing the health of the endogenous flora, can aid in reducing digestive upset caused by poor digestion of dietary fiber.

Enhancement of Epithelial Barrier Function

The intestinal epithelium forms the barrier between the outside of the body and the inside, much like your skin forms the barrier on the outside of your body. The integrity of the epithelium is crucial for preventing pathogens from entering the body. Intestinal barrier function relies on several defense mechanisms; antimicrobial peptides and secretory Immunoglobulin A (IgA) form a chemical barrier, while the mucous layer and the epithelial junction adhesion complex (i.e., tight junctions) form a physical barrier. Disruption of any of these layers of defense exposes the cells of the epithelium to bacterial and food antigens and can cause an inflammatory response. If this disruption becomes chronic it can lead to intestinal disorders such as IBS.

Probiotics have been shown to help repair a damaged epithelial barrier in several ways. First, they can suppress the inflammatory response by interacting with immune cells and alter inflammatory cytokine levels. Recently, it has been discovered that some probiotics can prevent inflammation-induced destruction of epithelial cells by preventing apoptosis. Probiotics can also alter gene expression of tight junction proteins, repairing the epithelial junction adhesion complex.

Some probiotics may also increase mucin secretion, thereby enhancing the mucosal barrier. Finally, in response to attack by pathogenic bacteria, probiotic strains can also induce the release of antimicrobial proteins from epithelial cells.

Increased Adhesion to Intestinal Mucosa or Inhibition of Pathogen Adhesion

There are a number of ways that probiotics have been shown to protect against the colonization of pathogenic bacteria (Bermudez-Brito et al. 2012). Inhibition of pathogen adhesion, competitive exclusion of pathogenic microorganisms, and production of antimicrobial substances are the primary ways in which probiotics can help protect us from colonization of pathogenic bacteria.

Adhesion of bacteria to mucosal surfaces and epithelial cells is one of the key beneficial features of probiotic action. Adhesion is a prerequisite for intestinal colonization and antagonistic activity against pathogenic bacteria. By this mechanism, endogenous intestinal bacteria as well as some probiotics supplements can provide competitive exclusion of potential pathogenic bacteria.

In part, competitive exclusion of pathogenic bacteria occurs by competitive inhibition of binding sites. Simply put, if you fill all the available binding sites with good bacteria, bad bacteria have nowhere to adhere and are left to continue their journey out of the body. Think of it like musical chairs for bacteria. When the music stops, some probiotics are good at grabbing the only available seats, leaving the bad guys with nowhere to sit. The importance of competitive exclusion becomes obvious when a broad-spectrum antibiotic therapy reduces the number of good bacteria and decreases colonization resistance, which may lead to an overgrowth of opportunistic pathogenic bacteria such as *Clostridium difficile* (Shanahan 2002).

Probiotics also release what are called autogenic regulation factors like lactic acid and hydrogen peroxide. These are antimicrobial substances that make the environment unfavorable for pathogenic bacteria to live. Some of these antimicrobial substances such as bacteriocides act directly to kill pathogenic bacteria.

Modulation of Immune Responses

Approximately 70 percent of the immune system is situated along the intestinal tract as gut-associated lymphoid tissue (GALT). This makes sense considering that the intestinal tract is the primary pathway for outside substances to enter the body. Many human studies have been performed to investigate the effects of probiotic cultures on the immune system. Some studies focused on the intestinal immune system, others on the systemic immunity, including allergies and juvenile asthma. These studies reveal that probiotic bacteria are able to enhance both innate and acquired immunity by increasing natural killer cell activity and phagocytosis, changing cytokine profiles, and increasing levels of immunoglobulins. The two most common species of probiotics *Bifidobacterium* and *Lactobacillus* have both been demonstrated in several studies to enhance natural immune function in healthy people as have most other common strains.

Safety

The long history of safety has contributed to the acceptance of probiotics as a safe food adjunct. Consequently, many probiotic products and their use in food products and dietary supplements have been granted GRAS status. GRAS status can be achieved when a probiotic has a history of safe use dating before 1958 or have been recognized by experts as safe under the conditions of intended use. For example, *B. coagulans* GBI-30-SF has had GRAS status since 2007 for general use as a probiotic. *B. animalis* subsp. *lactis* BB-12 and *S. thermophilus* TH-4 have had GRAS status since 2002 for specific use in infant formula.

The assumption of GRAS status however, has been frequently generalized for all probiotic strains being marketed in foods and dietary supplements. There are reported cases of probiotics from the genera *Lactobacillus, Leuconostoc, Pediococcus, Enterococcus*, and *Bifidobacterium* that have been isolated from infection sites, leading to the belief that these probiotics can translocate. Bacterial translocation is defined as the passage of viable bacteria (good or pathogenic) from the gastrointestinal tract to sites within the body outside of the gastrointestinal tract.

Commensal bacteria and probiotics have been identified in locations such as the mesenteric lymph node complex, liver, spleen, kidney, and bloodstream. The three primary mechanisms allowing bacterial translocation in animal models are: (a) disruption of the microbiota within the digestive tract leading to intestinal bacterial overgrowth, (b) increased permeability of the intestinal mucosal barrier, and (c) deficiencies in host immune defenses (Berg 1999).

Probiotic translocation is difficult to induce in healthy humans, and even if it does occur, detrimental effects are rare. Despite this, probiotics may still induce detrimental effects and various reports have documented health-damaging effects of probiotic translocation in immunocompromised patients. Due to probiotics' high degree of safety and their morphological confusion with other pathogenic bacteria, they are often overlooked as a potential risk and are least suspected as pathogens. Antibiotic resistance of some probiotic strains, however, has increased the complexity of treating infections in the immunocompromised individual (Liong 2008).

Glucosamine and Chondroitin

Background

Glucosamine and Chondroitin are naturally occurring chemical compounds that are found throughout the body, most notably in the extracellular matrix of the cartilage tissue of joints. The two compounds have clinical support for joint health benefits when used individually, but they are most commonly consumed in combination. The most common form of glucosamine found in dietary supplements is glucosamine sulfate, but glucosamine hydrochloride and n-acetyl glucosamine sources are also available. Glucosamine is most commonly sourced from the shells of shellfish, but it may be synthesized in a laboratory setting as well. Chondroitin is most commonly sourced as chondroitin sulfate. Chondroitin is comprised of repeating subunits of D-glucuronic acid and N-acetyl-D-galactosamine with sulfates attached to either the four- or six-position on the N-acetyl-D-galactosamine. When the sulfate resides in the four-position, the chondroitin is classified as CS A and when it falls in the six-position, it is classified as CS C. Chondroitin is most commonly sourced from bovine or porcine trachea and less commonly from avian sources.

Glucosamine and chondroitin are used by the body as substrates or building blocks in the formation of articular cartilage. Both ingredients have been shown to concentrate in the joint tissues following oral supplementation (Conte et al. 1995; Setnikar, Giacchetti, and Zanolo 1986; Setnikar et al. 1993). Glucosamine is specifically required for and is a rate-limiting step in the production of macromolecules found in articular cartilage, including proteoglycans, glycosaminoglycans, and hyaluronic acid. Glucosamine has also been found to have anti-inflammatory effects in the body (Gouze et al. 2002; Nakamura et al. 2004; Uitterlinden et al. 2006). Chondroitin is combined with proteins in the formation of proteoglycans, which provide structural resistance to compression forces in the joint, a key function of cartilage. The chondroitin compound is also a hydrophilic (water-loving) molecule, which attracts water into the cartilage, causing it to swell, and further supports this compression resistance quality (Bali, Cousse, and Neuzil 2001).

Rationale for Supplementation

Osteoarthritis (OA) affects millions of adults around the world, creating a worldwide public health problem. Symptoms of OA include pain, stiffness and reduced functionality. These effects often reduce quality of life for those individuals suffering from arthritis. Current treatment options include physical activity, hot and cold therapy, maintenance of a healthy weight, assistive devices, rest, and over-the-counter pain relievers or anti-inflammatory medications. In severe cases, joint replacement surgery may be necessary. Glucosamine and chondroitin at 1,500 and 1,200 mg/day, respectively, have been used alone and in combination by individuals with OA or age related declines in joint health and function. This supplement combination has been used for prevention and management of OA for almost 40 years (Vangsness, Spiker, and Erickson 2009).

Relief of joint pain and stiffness is the most common motivation for which consumers look to glucosamine and chondroitin supplementation. Clinical studies have shown that supplementation with glucosamine, chondroitin or the combination of the two can reduce these symptoms of OA over time. Significant improvements in pain, stiffness, and movement in subjects with OA have been demonstrated with glucosamine supplementation (Bruyere et al. 2004; Herrero-Beaumont et al. 2007; Pavelka et al. 2002; Reginster et al. 2001; Thie, Prasad, and Major 2001), chondroitin supplementation (Bourgeois et al. 1998; Bucsi and Poor 1998; Mazieres et al. 2007; Uebelhart et al. 2004), and a combination of the two (Clegg et al. 2006; Das and Hammad 2000; Leffler et al. 1999). The most notable study of this dietary supplement combination is the NIH-sponsored Glucosamine/Chondroitin Arthritis Intervention Trial (GAIT) (Clegg et al. 2006). This study included ~1,500 OA subjects and included five groups: 1,500 mg/day glucosamine hydrochloride, 1,200 mg/day chondroitin sulfate, the combination of the two, 200 mg/day of Celebrex™, or placebo. The study ran for 24 weeks. Significant improvements in pain were not found for the supplement groups versus placebo, but when results were controlled for those subjects with moderate to severe baseline pain, supplementation with glucosamine and chondroitin resulted in a significant improvement in pain versus placebo.

Another consequence of OA and aging on joint health is the steady breakdown of the cartilage matrix and its components. While the breakdown and rebuilding of cartilage is a natural process that occurs throughout life, during the aging process and OA, the balance between these two processes can shift away from one of cartilage building toward one of cartilage breakdown. Over time, this shift may result in a loss of cartilage thickness and a narrowing of the joint space. Supplementation with glucosamine and chondroitin has been found to support the structural integrity of cartilage and reduce its breakdown over time. In support of this benefit, 1,500 mg of glucosamine sulfate was shown in a clinical trial including 106 subjects with mild to moderate knee OA, to delay the progression of joint space narrowing compared with placebo over a 3-year period (Reginster et al. 2001). Similarly, several studies have shown that over time, supplementation with chondroitin sulfate at 800 mg or more per day results in a reduction in cartilage loss as compared to a placebo (Kahan, Reginster, and Vignon 2006; Michel et al. 2005; Uebelhart et al. 1998; Uebelhart et al. 2004; Wildi et al. 2011).

Given the previously referenced clinical evidence, individuals looking to support their overall joint health as they age may benefit from daily supplementation with 1,500 mg glucosamine and 1,200 mg chondroitin. Such supplementation may help reduce joint discomfort, improve flexibility, support healthy movement, and reduce age-related breakdown in articular cartilage. Furthermore, individuals taking Glucosamine may also be able to avoid or delay the need for knee replacement surgery. In 2007 researchers conducted a 5-year follow-up study of a group of knee OA patients who had participated in a clinical trial providing 1,500 mg of glucosamine sulfate. Results of this study demonstrated that those subjects who had supplemented with glucosamine for at least 12 months were 57 percent less likely to require a total knee replacement versus those subjects who had been taking a placebo (Bruyere et al. 2008).

Safety

Glucosamine and Chondroitin are likely safe when taken orally by healthy adults at or below the most commonly recommended dosages of 1,500 and 1,200 mg daily, respectively. DRIs for these compounds have not been determined; therefore, adequate intake levels and tolerable upper limits do not exist for these ingredients. Few studies have been conducted to evaluate the safety of glucosamine or chondroitin at doses that exceed the recommended levels of 1,500 and 1,200 mg/day, respectively. Glucosamine is derived from shrimp, crab, and other shellfish, and consequently should be avoided by individuals with an allergy or sensitivity to shellfish or iodine. Some research has linked glucosamine intake with increased blood sugar levels, while other studies have not found the same result; so individuals with diabetes should consult their physician before considering taking this supplement (Anderson, Nicolosi, and Borzelleca 2005; Biggee et al. 2007; Muniyappa et al. 2006; Scroggie, Albright, and Harris 2003; Tannis, Barban, and Conquer 2004). Chondroitin may increase an individual's risk for bleeding. Individuals with bleeding disorders should consult their physician before taking chondroitin. As with all dietary supplements, individuals with any diseases or medical conditions should consult their physician before taking any dietary supplements.

Coenzyme Q10

Background

Coenzyme Q10 (also known as ubiquinone, ubidecarenone, or CoQ10) is a lipid-soluble vitamin-like compound both synthesized in the body and consumed in the diet. CoQ10 is present in the inner membrane of the mitochondria of every cell of the body. The name ubiquinone refers to the ubiquitous presence of these compounds in living organisms and their chemical structure, which contains a functional group known as a benzoquinone. The structure of CoQ10 consists of a benzoquinone ring and a lipophilic isoprenoid side chain. The length of the side chain varies, but in humans, the side chain is composed of 10 trans-isoprenoid units, thus coenzyme Q "10."

CoQ10 plays two major roles in the body. In the mitochondria, CoQ10 is a vital coenzyme in the electron transport chain for the synthesis of ATP, the major source of cellular energy. CoQ10 is found at its highest levels in cells with high energy requirements such as heart, brain, liver, and kidney. The second function of CoQ10 is as an antioxidant, particularly in preventing lipid peroxidation. CoQ10 also plays a role in the regeneration of other antioxidants. CoQ10 bears a close relationship with vitamin E allowing it to regenerate in its active, reduced form (alpha-tocopherol). It also serves in the regeneration of the reduced form of vitamin C (ascorbate).

Although CoQ10 is not classified as an essential nutrient, low tissue and serum levels of CoQ10 have been associated with a number of conditions including cardiovascular disease, neuromuscular conditions, hypertension, periodontal disease, asthma, hyperthyroidism, male infertility, and AIDS. CoQ10 deficiency could result from reduced CoQ10 synthesis secondary to other nutritional deficiencies, a genetic or acquired defect in CoQ10 synthesis or utilization, or a conditional deficiency due to increased tissue needs associated with a specific illness. CoQ10 has been used in experimental settings as a treatment for these conditions with varying success. Outcomes suffer from variable serum levels within each subject. This has been attributed in part to the poor bioavailability of common CoQ10 supplements (Bank, Kagan, and Madhavi 2011).

Bioavailability of CoQ10

CoQ10 is a lipid-soluble compound with a high molecular weight (864 Daltons), and this fact can limit absorption. CoQ10 absorption is known to improve in the presence of fat, thus dietary supplements containing powdered CoQ10 formulations that are suspended or emulsified in oil are better absorbed than the powder alone. CoQ10 emulsified in oil will come in the form of a softgel, not a two piece capsule. Many other technologies or systems have been investigated for their ability to enhance absorption. Examples include solubilized formulations in emulsifiers such as soy lecithin, polysorbates, and medium-chain triglycerides. Micronization of raw crystalline CoQ10 powder is often used in these formulations as is micellarization and are often blended with absorption enhancers. CoQ10 can also be complexed with cyclodextrins to form a water-soluble compound. Other formulations include colloidal and nano-beadlet delivery systems (Bank, Kagan, and Madhavi 2011).

Marketers of CoQ10 supplements seek after and rely heavily on the "enhanced absorption" claim on their packaging. Comparative studies looking at bioavailability show that these delivery systems differ, sometimes significantly, in their capacity to improve bioavailability. One must also be aware that most of the studies comparing bioavailability of CoQ10 formulations are conducted or sponsored by companies with a financial interest in the outcome of the study. This does not guarantee that bias is playing a factor in the outcome, but it is always a possibility and is more likely when studies are sponsored by manufactures. Consequently, if there is a quantitative claim about just how much better it is absorbed, take it with a grain of salt, as different absorption technologies and testing methods will return different results.

In addition to formulas designed to enhance the absorption of CoQ10 (ubiquinone), another form of CoQ10 referred to as ubiquin-*ol* is also sold as a dietary supplement. Ubiquinol is claimed to have superior bioavailability. Ubiquinone is the form synthesized in the body's cells. It is then converted to ubiquinol. Ubiquinone is the oxidized form of CoQ10, and ubiquinol is the reduced form, and together they form a redox pair. Each can be readily converted into the other in cells, lymph, or the blood when their respective forms are needed. Ingested CoQ10 in the foods we eat is converted to ubiquinone upon cooking. Likewise, ubiquinol ingested as a dietary supplement is converted to ubiquinone in the stomach. Ubiquinol is only slightly more water soluble than ubiquinone. Ubiquinol is considerably more expensive than ubiquinone and the many forms of Ubiquinone (CoQ10) (aside from dry powder) have many years of data demonstrating their effectiveness, so ubiquinone as CoQ10 is generally considered the best option for the majority of consumers.

Rationale for Supplementation

The most common reason people take CoQ10 is for general wellness. CoQ10 is important for the proper functioning of every tissue in the body due to its role in cellular energy production and antioxidant activity. Secondary reasons most often include antiaging and heart health.

Antiaging

Theories explaining the mechanism of aging include the mitochondrial theory of aging. This theory proposes that progressive accumulation of mutations in mitochondrial DNA during our lifetime leads to a decline in mitochondrial function. This is postulated as a key contributing factor to human aging (Wei et al. 2009). CoQ10 levels decline with advancing age, and this decline might play a role in the increase in mitochondrial mutations and declining function of mitochondria. To date, dietary CoQ10 supplementation has not shown direct effects on extending life span in animal studies. Thus, it may be considered that dietary CoQ10 supplementation may not directly extend lifespan; however it may help to prevent life span *shortening* due to cellular oxidative damage (López-Lluch et al. 2010). One possible exception in which anti-aging effects *have* been seen is in the beneficial effects of CoQ10 treatment on non–disease-related skin aging (Prahl et al. 2008).

Heart Health

CoQ10 has been investigated as a potential therapy for a large number of health conditions and diseases, especially those that result from reduced mitochondrial function. Currently, CoQ10 is widely promoted as a dietary supplement for supporting cardiovascular health. Myocardial cells contain some of the highest concentrations of CoQ10 in the body (Kumar et al. 2009). The cardiovascular benefits of CoQ10 have been credited to its role in ATP production, its capability of antagonizing oxidation of LDL-cholesterol, its regulation of cell membrane channels, and its ability to reduce the effects of endothelial damage, specifically by improving endothelial function (Mortensen 2003; Sinatra 2009). Consequently, much attention has been directed toward therapies that promote and maintain ATP production.

One aspect of coronary heart failure is ATP consumption exceeding ATP production, resulting in oxidative stress. Patients with heart failure and cardiomyopathy have decreased plasma CoQ10. CoQ10 supplementation can increase left ventricular ejection fraction by as much as 22 to 39 percent in patients with coronary heart failure. Interestingly it also increased ejection fraction by 4 percent in healthy subjects (Langsjoen and Langsjoen 2008; Molyneux et al. 2008). In addition, supplemental CoQ10 increased walking tolerance and decreased distal limb edema in this population. Finally, Molyneux et al. (2008) observed that serum CoQ10 values were an independent predictor of mortality, thereby supporting the strategy of administering CoQ10 to this group.

Effects of CoQ10 Supplementation on Blood Pressure

Studies have shown CoQ10 can lower arterial blood pressure in individuals with hypertension (Wyman, Leonard, and Morledge 2010). The exact mechanism is not known, but one theory suggests it reduces peripheral resistance by increasing peripheral endothelial function (Pepe et al. 2007). Wyman, Leonard, and Morledge (2010) suggested CoQ10 may increase the production of nitric oxide and prostaglandin prostacyclin, both potent vasodilators and inhibitors of platelet aggregation. It should be noted however that in healthy humans and animals CoQ10 has not been shown to possess a direct vasodilating or acute hypotensive effect. This indicates that the hypotensive effect of CoQ10 is likely to be specific to the state of enhanced oxidative stress occurring in hypertensive individuals (Rosenfeldt et al. 2007).

Studies examining the efficacy of CoQ10 as an adjunct to treat essential hypertension are conflicting, in part due to variations in the methods of administering CoQ10 and in part to the study design adopted (Ho, Bellusci, and Wright 2009). Digiesi Cantini and Brodbeck (1990) studied 18 patients with essential hypertension. Patients were randomized to receive either 100 mg/day of CoQ10 or a placebo for 10 weeks. This study ensured the effects were linked specifically to CoQ10 by discontinuing antihypertensive therapy prior to the study. The patients receiving CoQ10 exhibited significant decreases in systolic and diastolic pressures at 3 weeks of treatment, which persisted throughout the subsequent 7 weeks of treatment. After 10 weeks, CoQ10 administration was stopped, resulting in blood pressures increasing to pretreatment levels in 7 to 10 days. A meta-analysis of 12 clinical trials concluded CoQ10 lowered systolic blood pressure by up to 17 mm Hg and diastolic blood pressure by up to 10 mm Hg in patients with essential hypertension without any significant side effects (Rosenfeldt et al. 2007).

Still, not all studies looking at the effects of CoQ10 on blood pressure have demonstrated a clear benefit. A recent 12-week randomized double-blind placebo controlled crossover study by Young et al. (2012) administered CoQ10 or placebo to 30 subjects with the metabolic syndrome (i.e., prediabetes) while maintaining their conventional blood pressure drug regimen. Compared with placebo, CoQ10 was not associated with a statistically significant reduction in blood pressure. These findings concur with one other double-blind, placebo-controlled intervention trial by Mori et al. (2009), who found 8 weeks of CoQ10 administration had no effect on 24-hour ambulatory blood pressure in patients with chronic kidney disease. Interestingly, Young reported that although no significant difference was found for 24-hour measures of blood pressure, daytime "diastolic BP loads" were significantly lower while taking CoQ10 (Young et al. 2012).

Safety

CoQ10 supplementation is GRAS. There is a paucity of adverse events reported in short and long term human and animal studies. The most common complaints are stomach upset, but this is associated with three or more g/day. Long term, CoQ10 has been safely used in studies lasting up to 30 months.

References

Anderson, J.W., P. Baird, R.H. Davis Jr, S. Ferreri, M. Knudtson, A. Koraym, V. Waters, and C.L. Williams. 2009. "Health Benefits of Dietary Fiber." *Nutrition Reviews* 67, no. 4, pp. 188–205. doi:10.1111/j.1753-4887.2009.00189.x

Anderson, J.W., R.J. Nicolosi, and J.F. Borzelleca. 2005. "Glucosamine Effects in Humans: A Review of Effects on Glucose Metabolism, Side Effects, Safety Considerations and Efficacy." *Food and Chemical Toxicology* 43, no. 2, pp. 187–201. doi:10.1016/j.fct.2004.11.006

Appleton, K.M., R.C. Hayward, D. Gunnell, T.J. Peters, P.J. Rogers, D. Kessler, and A.R. Ness. 2006. "Effects of n-3 Long-Chain Polyunsaturated Fatty Acids on Depressed Mood: Systematic Review of Published Trials." *American Journal of Clinical Nutrition* 84, no. 6, pp. 1308–16.

Backhed, F., R.E. Ley, J.L. Sonnenburg, D.A. Peterson, and J.I. Gordon. 2005. "Host-Bacterial Mutualism in the Human Intestine." *Science* 307, no. 5717, pp. 1915–20. doi:10.1126/science.1104816

Bali, J.P., H. Cousse, and E. Neuzil. 2001. "Biochemical Basis of the Pharmacologic Action of Chondroitin Sulfates on the Osteoarticular System." *Seminars in Arthritis Rheumatism* 31, no. 1, pp. 58–68. doi:10.1053/sarh.2000.24874

Bank, G., D. Kagan, and D. Madhavi. 2011. "Coenzyme Q10: Clinical Update and Bioavailability." *Journal of Evidence-Based Complementary & Alternative Medicine* 129. doi:10.1177/2156587211399438

Berg, R.D. 1999. "Bacterial Translocation from the Gastrointestinal Tract." *Advances in Experimental Medicine and Biology*, pp. 11–30. doi:10.1007/978-1-4615-4143-1_2

Bermudez-Brito, M., J. Plaza-Díaz, S. Muñoz-Quezada, C. Gómez-Llorente, and A. Gil. 2012. "Probiotic Mechanisms of Action." *Annuals of Nutrition and Metabolism* 61, no. 2, pp. 160–74. doi:10.1159/000342079

Biggee, B.A., C.M. Blinn, M. Nuite, J.E. Silbert, and T.E. McAlindon. 2007. "Effects of Oral Glucosamine Sulphate on Serum Glucose and Insulin During an Oral Glucose Tolerance Test of Subjects with Osteoarthritis." *Annuals of Rheumatic Disease* 66, no. 2, pp. 260–62. doi:10.1136/ard.2006.058222

Blasbalg, T.L., T.L. Blasbalg, J.R. Hibbeln, C.E. Ramsden, S.F. Majchrzak, and R.R. Rawlings. 2011. "Changes in Consumption of Omega-3 and Omega-6 Fatty Acids in the United States During the 20th Century." *American Journal of Clinical Nutrition* 93, no. 5, pp. 950–62. doi:10.3945/ajcn.110.006643

Bloch, M.H., and Q. Ahmad. 2011. "Omega-3 Fatty Acid Supplementation for the Treatment of Children with Attention-Deficit/Hyperactivity Disorder Symptomatology: Systematic Review and Meta-Analysis." *Journal of the American Academy of Child and Adolescent Psychiatry* 50, no. 10, pp. 991–1000. doi:10.1016/j.jaac.2011.06.008

Bottino, N.V. 1957. "Resistance of Certain Long-Chain Polyunsaturated Fatty Acids of Marine Oils to Pancreatic Lipase Hydrolysis." *Lipids* 2, no. 6, pp. 489–93. doi:10.1007/bf02533177

Bourgeois, P., G. Chales, J. Dehais, B. Delcambre, J.L. Kuntz, and S. Rozenberg. 1998. "Efficacy and Tolerability of Chondroitin Sulfate 1200 mg/day vs Chondroitin Sulfate 3 × 400 mg/day vs Placebo." *Osteoarthritis Cartilage* 6 Suppl A, pp. 25–30. doi:10.1016/s1063-4584(98)80008-3

Broughton, K.S., C.S. Johnson, B.K. Pace, M. Liebman, and K.M. Kleppinger. 1997. "Reduced Asthma Symptoms with n–3 Fatty Acid Ingestion are Related to 5-Series Leukotriene Production." *American Journal of Clinical Nutrition* 65, no. 4, pp. 1011–17.

Bruyere, O., K. Pavelka, L.C. Rovati, J. Gatterova, G. Giacovelli, M. Olejarova, R. Deroisy, and J.Y. Reginster. 2008. "Total Joint Replacement after Glucosamine Sulphate Treatment in Knee Osteoarthritis: Results of a Mean 8-Year Observation of Patients from Two Previous 3-Year, Randomised, Placebo-Controlled Trials." *Osteoarthritis and Cartilage* 16, no. 2, pp. 254–60. doi:10.1016/j.joca.2007.06.011

Bruyere, O., K. Pavelka, L.C. Rovati, R. Deroisy, M. Olejarova, J. Gatterova, G. Giacovelli, and J.Y. Reginster. 2004. "Glucosamine Sulfate Reduces Osteoarthritis Progression in Postmenopausal Women with Knee Osteoarthritis: Evidence from Two 3-Year Studies." *Menopause* 11, no. 2, pp. 138–43. doi:10.1097/01.gme.0000087983.28957.5d

Bucsi, L., and G. Poor. 1998. "Efficacy and Tolerability of Oral Chondroitin Sulfate as a Symptomatic Slow-Acting Drug for Osteoarthritis (SYSADOA) in the Treatment of Knee Osteoarthritis." *Osteoarthritis Cartilage* 6 Suppl A, pp. 31–36. doi:10.1016/s1063-4584(98)80009-5

Clegg, D.O., D.J. Reda, C.L. Harris, M.A. Klein, J.R. O'Dell, M.M. Hooper, J.D. Bradley, C.O. Bingham 3rd, M.H. Weisman, C.G. Jackson, N.E. Lane, J.J. Cush, L.W. Moreland, H.R. Schumacher Jr., C.V. Oddis, F. Wolfe, J.A. Molitor, D.E. Yocum, T.J. Schnitzer, D.E. Furst, A.D. Sawitzke, H. Shi, K.D. Brandt, R.W. Moskowitz, and H.J. Williams. 2006. "Glucosamine, Chondroitin Sulfate, and the Two in Combination for Painful Knee Osteoarthritis." *New England Journal of Medicine* 354, no. 8, pp. 795–808. doi:10.1056/NEJMoa052771

Conte, A., N. Volpi, L. Plamieri, I. Bahous, and G. Ronca. 1995. "Biochemical and Pharmacokinetic Aspects of Oral Treatment with Chondroitin Sulfate." *Arzneimittelforschung* 45, no. 8, pp. 918–25.

Coussement, P.A. 1999. "Inulin and Oligofructose: Safe Intakes and Legal Status." *The Journal of Nutrition* 129, no. 7, pp. 1412S–7S.

da Rocha, C.M., and K. Gilberto. 2012. "High Dietary Ratio of Omega-6 to Omega-3 Polyunsaturated Acids during Pregnancy and Prevalence of Post-Partum Depression." *Maternal Child Nutrition* 8, no. 1, pp. 36–48. doi:10.1111/j.1740-8709.2010.00256.x

Danaei, G., E.L. Ding, D. Mozaffarian, B. Taylor, J. Rehm, C.J.L. Murray, and M. Ezzati. 2009. "The Preventable Causes of Death in the United States: Comparative Risk Assessment of Dietary, Lifestyle, and Metabolic Risk Factors." *PLoS Medicine* 6, no. 4: e1000058. doi:10.1371/journal.pmed.1000058

Das, A., Jr., and T.A. Hammad. 2000. "Efficacy of a Combination of FCHG49 Glucosamine Hydrochloride, TRH122 Low Molecular Weight Sodium Chondroitin Sulfate and Manganese Ascorbate in the Management of Knee Osteoarthritis." *Osteoarthritis and Cartilage* 8, no. 5, pp. 343–50. doi:10.1053/joca.1999.0308

Dash, S.K. 2009. "Selection Criteria for Probiotics." *XXXVII Dairy Industry Conference.* Panjim, India: Kala Academy.

Deutsch, L. 2007. "Evaluation of the Effect of Neptune Krill Oil on Chronic Inflammation and Arthritic Symptoms." *Journal of the American College of Nutrition* 26, no. 1, pp. 39–48. doi:10.1080/07315724.2007.10719584

Digiesi, V., F. Cantini, and B. Brodbeck. 1990. "Effect of Coenzyme Q10 on Essential Arterial Hypertension." *Current Therapeutic Research* 47, no. 5, pp. 841–45.

DiNicolantonio, J.J., A.K. Niazi, M.F. McCarty, J.H. O'Keefe, P. Meier, and C.J. Lavie. 2014. "Omega-3s and Cardiovascular Health." *The Ochsner Journal* 14, no. 3, pp. 399–412.

FAO/WHO. 2001. Evaluation of Health and Properties of Probiotics in Food Including Powder Milk with Live Lactic Acid Bacteria. Joint FAO/WHO Expert Consultation, Córdoba, Argentina: FAO/WHO.

Flock, M.R., A.C. Skulas-Ray, W.S. Harris, T.D. Etherton, J.A. Fleming, and P.M. Kris-Etherton. 2013. "Determinants of Erythrocyte Omega-3 Fatty Acid Content in Response to Fish Oil Supplementation: A Dose-Response Randomized Controlled Trial." *Journal of the American Heart Association* 2, no. 6: e000513. doi:10.1161/jaha.113.000513

Fortin, P.R., R.A. Lew, M.H. Liang, E.A. Wright, L.A. Beckett, T.C. Chalmers, and R.I. Sperling. 1995. "Validation of a Meta-Analysis: The Effects of Fish Oil in Rheumatoid Arthritis." *Journal of Clinical Epidemiology* 48, no. 11, pp. 1379–90. doi:10.1016/0895-4356(95)00028-3

Garaiova, I., I.A. Guschina, S.F. Plummer, J. Tang, D. Wang, and N.T. Plummer. 2007. "A Randomized Cross-Over Trial in Healthy Adults Indicating Improved Absorption of Omega-3 Fatty Acids by Pre-Emulsification." *Nutrition Journal* 6, p. 4. doi:10.1186/1475-2891-6-4

Gibson, G.R., and M.B. Roberfroid. 1995. "Dietary Modulation of the Human Colonic Microbiota: Introducing the Concept of Prebiotics." *Journal of Nutrition* 125, no. 6, pp. 1401–12.

Gibson, G.R., K.P. Scott, R.A. Rastall, K.M. Tuohy, A. Hotchkiss, A. Dubert-Ferrandon, M. Gareau, E.F. Murphy, D. Saulnier, G. Loh, S. Macfarlane, N. Delzenne, Y. Ringel, G. Kozianowski, R. Dickmann, I. Lenoir-Wijnkoop, C. Walker, and R. Buddington. 2010. "Dietary Prebiotics: Current Status and New Definition." *Food Science and Technology Bulletin: Functional Foods* 7, no. 1, pp. 1–19. doi:10.1616/1476-2137.15880

Gillies, D., J.K. Sinn, S.S. Lad, M.J. Leach, and M.J. Ross. 2012. "Polyunsaturated Fatty Acids (PUFA) for Attention Deficit Hyperactivity Disorder (ADHD) in Children and Adolescents." *Cochrane Database of Systematic Reviews*, no. 7: CD007986. doi:10.1002/14651858.CD007986.pub2

Goktepe, I., V.K. Juneja, and M. Ahmedna. 2006. *Probiotics in Food Safety and Human Health.* Boca Raton, FL: CRC Press.

Goldberg, R.J., and J. Katz. 2007. "A Meta-Analysis of the Analgesic Effects of Omega-3 Polyunsaturated Fatty Acidsupplementation for Inflammatory Joint Pain." *Pain* 129, no. 1, pp. 210–23. doi:10.1016/j.pain.2007.01.020

Gouze, J.N., A. Bianchi, P. Becuwe, M. Dauca, P. Netter, J. Magdalou, B. Terlain, and K. Bordji. 2002. "Glucosamine Modulates IL-1-Induced Activation of Rat Chondrocytes at a Receptor Level, and by Inhibiting the NF-Kappa B Pathway." *FEBS Letters* 510, no. 3, pp. 166–170. doi:10.1016/s0014-5793(01)03255-0

Harris, W.S., and C. von Schacky. 2004. "The Omega-3 Index: A New Risk Factor for Death from Coronary Heart Disease?" *Preventive Medicine* 39, no. 1, pp. 212–20. doi:10.1016/j.ypmed.2004.02.030

Harris, W. January 2015. "The Association of Red Blood Cell Omega-3 Fatty Acids (O3I) and Cardiovascular Risk." *The Omega-3 Index.* New York, NY: Presented at the meeting of the Global Nutrition and Health Alliance.

Helland, I.B., L. Smith, B. Blomen, K. Saarem, O.D. Saugstad, and C.A. Drevon. 2008. "Effect of Supplementing Pregnant and Lactating Mothers with n-3 Very-Long-Chain Fatty Acids on Children's IQ and Body Mass Index at 7 years of Age." *Pediatrics* 122, no. 2, pp. e472–79. doi:10.1542/peds.2007-2762

Helland, I.B., L. Smith, K. Saarem, O.D. Saugstad, and C.A. Drevon. 2003. "Maternal Supplementation with Very-Long-Chain n-3 Fatty Acids during Pregnancy and Lactation Augments Children's IQ at 4 Years of Age." *Pediatrics* 111, no. 1, pp. e39–44. doi:10.1542/peds.111.1.e39

Herrero-Beaumont, G., J.A. Ivorra, M. Del Carmen Trabado, F.J. Blanco, P. Benito, E. Martin-Mola, J. Paulino, J.L. Marenco, A. Porto, A. Laffon, D. Araujo, M. Figueroa, and J. Branco. 2007. "Glucosamine Sulfate in the Treatment of Knee Osteoarthritis Symptoms: A Randomized, Double-Blind, Placebo-Controlled Study Using Acetaminophen as a Side Comparator." *Arthritis & Rheumatism* 56, no. 2, pp. 555–67. doi:10.1002/art.22371

Hibbeln, J. 1998. "Fish Consumption and Major Depression." *Lancet* 351, no. 9110, p. 1213. doi:10.1016/s0140-6736(05)79168-6

Ho, M.J., A. Bellusci, and J.M. Wright. 2009. "Blood Pressure Lowering Efficacy of Coenzyme 010 for Primary Hypertension." *Cochrane Database Systematic Review* 7, no. 4: CD007435. doi:10.1002/14651858.cd007435.pub2

Hussein, N. 2005. "Long-Chain Conversion of [13C]Linoleic Acid and Alpha-Linolenic Acid in Response to Marked Changes in Their Dietary Intake in Men. *The Journal of Lipid Research* 46, no. 2, pp. 269–80. doi:10.1194/jlr.m400225-jlr200

Imhoff-Kunsch, B., V. Briggs, T. Goldenberg, and U. Ramakrishnan. 2012. "Effect of n-3 Long-Chain Polyunsaturated Fatty Acid Intake During Pregnancy on Maternal, Infant, and Child Health Outcomes: A Systematic Review." *Paediatr Perinat Epidemiol* 26, pp. 91–107. doi:10.1111/j.1365-3016.2012.01292.x

Jones, J.R., D.M. Lineback, and M.J. Levine. 2006. "Dietary Reference Intakes: Implications for Fiber Labeling and Consumption: A Summary of the International Life Sciences Institute North American FiberWorkshop 2004." *Nutrition Reviews* 64, no. 1, pp. 31–38. doi:10.1111/j.1753-4887.2006.tb00170.x

Kahan, A., J.Y. Reginster, and E. Vignon. 2006. "STOPP (Study on Osteoarthritis Progression Prevention): A New Two-Year Trial with Chondroitin 4 & 6 Sulfate (CS) [abstract]." In *EULAR*. The Netherlands, Amsterdam: Institut Biochimique SA.

Kendall, C., A. Esfahani, and D. Jenkins. 2010. "The Link Between Dietary Fibre and Human Health." *Food Hydrocolloids* 24, no. 1, pp. 42–48. doi:10.1016/j.foodhyd.2009.08.002

Kumar, A., H. Kaur, P. Devi, and V. Mohan. 2009. "Role of Coenzyme 010 (CoO10) in Cardiac Disease, Hypertension and Meniere-like Syndrome." *Pharmacology & Therapeutics* 124, no. 3, pp. 259–68. doi:10.1016/j.pharmthera.2009.07.003

Langsjoen, P.H., and A.M. Langsjoen. 2008. "Supplemental Ubiquinol in Patients with Advanced Congestive Heart Failure." *Biofactors* 32, no. 1–4, pp. 119–128. doi:10.1002/biof.5520320114

Leffler, C.T., A.F. Philippi, S.G. Leffler, J.C. Mosure, and P.D. Kim. 1999. "Glucosamine, Chondroitin, and Manganese Ascorbate for Degenerative Joint Disease of the Knee or Low Back: A Randomized, Double-Blind, Placebo-Controlled Pilot Study." *Military Medicine* 164, no. 2, pp. 85–91.

Lilly, D.M., and R.H. Stillwell. 1965. "Probiotics: Growth Promoting Factors Produced by Microorganisms." *Science* 147, no. 3659, pp. 747–48. doi:10.1126/science.147.3659.747

Lin, P.Y., and K. Su. 2007. "A Meta-Analytic Review of Double-Blind, Placebo-Controlled Trials of Antidepressant Efficacy of Omega-3 Fatty Acids." *Journal of Clinical Psychiatry* 68, no. 7, pp. 1056–61. doi:10.4088/jcp.v68n0712

Liong, M.T. 2008. "Safety of Probiotics: Translocation and Infection." *Nutrition Reviews* 66, no. 4, pp. 192–202. doi:10.1111/j.1753-4887.2008.00024.x

Liu, A., Y. Lin, R. Terry, K. Nelson, and P.S. Bernstein. 2011. "Role of Long-Chain and Very-Long-Chain Polyunsaturated Fatty Acids in Macular Degenerations and Dystrophies." *Clinical Lipidology* 6, no. 5, pp. 593–613. doi:10.2217/clp.11.41

López-Lluch, G., J.C. Rodríguez-Aguilera, C. Santos-Ocaña, and P. Navas. 2010. "Is Coenzyme Q a Key Factor in Aging?" *Mechanisms of Ageing and Development* 131, no. 4, pp. 225–35. doi:10.1016/j.mad.2010.02.003

Mas, E., K.D. Croft, P. Zahra, A. Barden, and T.A. Mori. 2012. "Resolvins D1, D2, and Other Mediators of Self-Limited Resolution of Inflammation in Human Blood Following n-3 Fatty Acid Supplementation." *Clinical Chemistry* 58, no. 10, pp. 1476–84. doi:10.1373/clinchem.2012.190199

Mazieres, B., M. Hucher, M. Zaim, and P. Garnero. 2007. "Effect of Chondroitin Sulphate in Symptomatic Knee Osteoarthritis: A Multicentre, Randomised, Double-Blind, Placebo-Controlled Study." *Annuals of Rheumatic Diseases* 66, no. 5, pp. 639–45. doi:10.1136/ard.2006.059899

McRorie, J.W., Jr. 2015a. "Evidence-Based Approach to Fiber Supplements and Clinically Meaningful Health Benefits, Part 1: What to Look for and How to Recommend an Effective Fiber Therapy." *Nutrition Today* 50, no. 2, pp. 82–89. doi:10.1097/nt.0000000000000082

McRorie, J.W., Jr. 2015b. "Evidence-Based Approach to Fiber Supplements and Clinically Meaningful Health Benefits, Part 2: What to Look for and How to Recommend an Effective Fiber Therapy." *Nutrition Today* 50, no. 2, pp. 90–97. doi:10.1097/nt.00000000000000829

Melanson, S.F., E.L. Lewandrowski, J.G. Flood, and K.B. Lewandrowski. 2005. "Measurement of Organochlorines in Commercial Over-the-Counter Fish Oil Preparations: Implications for Dietary and Therapeutic Recommendations for Omega-3 Fatty Acids and a Review of the Literature." *Archives of Pathology & Laboratory Medicine* 129, no. 1, pp. 74–77.

Metchnikoff, E. 1907. "Lactic Acid as Inhibiting Intestinal Putrefaction." In *The Prolongation of Life: Optimistic Studies*, ed. E. Metchnikoff, 161–83. London, UK: G.P. Putnam's Sons.

Michel, B.A., G. Stucki, D. Frey, F. De Vathaire, E. Vignon, P. Bruehlmann, and D. Uebelhart. 2005. "Chondroitins 4 and 6 Sulfate in Osteoarthritis of the Knee: A Randomized, Controlled Trial." *Arthritis & Rheumatism* 52, no. 3, pp. 779–86. doi:10.1002/art.20867

Molendi-Coste, O., V. Legry, and I.A. Leclercq. 2011. "Why and How Meet n-3 PUFA Dietary Recommendations?" *Gastroenterology Research and Practice* 2011, pp. 1–11: 364040. doi:10.1155/2011/364040

Molyneux, S.L., C.M. Florkowski, P.M. George, A.P. Pilbrow, C.M. Frampton, M. Lever, and A.M. Richards. 2008. "Coenzyme Q10: An Independent Predictor of Mortality in Chronic Heart Failure." *Journal of the American College of Cardiology* 52, no. 18, pp. 1435–41. doi:10.1016/j.jacc.2008.07.044

Mori, T.A., V. Burke, I. Puddey, A. Irish, C.A. Cowpland, L. Beilin, G. Dogra, and G.F. Watts. 2009. "The Effects of [omega]3 fatty Acids and Coenzyme Q10 on Blood Pressure and Heart Rate in Chronic Kidney Disease: A Randomized Controlled Trial." *Journal of Hypertension* 27, no. 9, pp. 1863–72. doi:10.1097/hjh.0b013e32832e1bd9

Mortensen, S.A. 2003. "Overview on Coenzyme O10 as Adjunctive Therapy in Chronic Heart Failure. Rationale, Design and Endpoints of "Q-symbio" - A Multinational Trial." *Biofactors* 18, no. 1–4, pp. 79–89. doi:10.1002/biof.5520180210

Muniyappa, R., R.J. Karne, G. Hall, S.K. Crandon, J.A. Bronstein, M.R. Ver, G.L. Hortin, and M.J. Quon. 2006. "Oral Glucosamine for 6 Weeks at Standard Doses Does Not Cause or Worsen Insulin Resistance or Endothelial Dysfunction in Lean or Obese Subjects." *Diabetes* 55, no. 1, pp. 3142–50. doi:10.2337/db06-0714

Nakamura, H., A. Shibakawa, M. Tanaka, T. Kato, and K. Nishioka. 2004. "Effects of Glucosamine Hydrochloride on the Production of Prostaglandin E2, Nitric Oxide and Metalloproteases by Chondrocytes and Synoviocytes in Osteoarthritis." *Clinical and Experimental Rheumatology* 22, no. 3, pp. 293–99.

Patrick, R.P., and B.N. Ames. 2015. "Vitamin D and the Omega-3 Fatty Acids Control Serotonin Synthesis and Action, Part 2: Relevance for ADHD, Bipolar, Schizophrenia, and Impulsive Behavior." *The FASEB Journal* 29, no. 6, pp. 2207–22. doi:10.1096/fj.14-268342

Patterson, E., R. Wall, G.F. Fitzgerald, R.P. Ross, and C. Stanton. 2012. "Health Implications of High Dietary Omega-6 Polyunsaturated Fatty Acids." *Journal of Nutrition Metabolism* 12, pp. 1–6: 539426. doi:10.1155/2012/539426

Pavelka, K., J. Gatterova, M. Olejarova, S. Machacek, G. Giacovelli, and L.C. Rovati. 2002. "Glucosamine Sulfate Use and Delay of Progression of Knee Osteoarthritis: A 3-Year, Randomized, Placebo-Controlled, Double-Blind Study." *Archives of Internal Medicine* 162, no. 18, pp. 2113–23. doi:10.1001/archinte.162.18.2113

Pepe, S., S.F. Marasco, S.J. Haas, F.L. Sheeran, H. Krum, and F.L. Rosenfeldt. 2007. "Coenzyme 010 in Cardiovascular Disease." *Mitochondrion* 7, pp. S154–167. doi:10.1016/j.mito.2007.02.005

Prahl, S., T. Kueper, T. Biernoth, Y. Wöhrmann, A. Münster, M. Fürstenau, M. Schmidt, C. Schulze, K.P. Wittern, H. Wenck, G.M. Muhr, and T. Blatt. 2008. "Aging Skin Is Functionally Anaerobic: Importance of Coenzyme Q10 for Anti-Aging Skin Care." *Biofactors* 32, no. 1–4, pp. 245–55. doi:10.1002/biof.5520320129

Raatz, S.K., J. Bruce Redmon, N. Wimmergren, J.V. Donadio, and D.M. Bibus. 2009. "Enhanced Absorption of n-3 Fatty Acids from Emulsified Compared with Encapsulated Fish Oil." *Journal of American Dietetic Association* 109, no. 6, pp. 1076–81. doi:10.1016/j.jada.2009.03.006

Reginster, J.Y., R. Deroisy, L.C. Rovati, R.L. Lee, E. Lejeune, O. Bruyere, G. Giacovelli, Y. Henrotin, J. E. Dacre, and C. Gossett. 2001. "Long-Term Effects of Glucosamine Sulphate on Osteoarthritis Progression: A Randomised, Placebo-Controlled Clinical Trial." *Lancet* 357, no. 9252, pp. 251–56. doi:10.1016/S0140-6736(00)03610-2

Roberfroid, M., G.R. Gibson, L. Hoyles, A.L. McCartney, R. Rastall, I. Rowland, D. Wolvers, B. Watzl, H. Szajewska, B. Stahl, F. Guarner, F. Respondek, K. Whelan, V. Coxam, M.-J. Davicco, L. Léotoing, Y. Wittrant, N.M. Delzenne, P.D. Cani, A.M. Neyrinck, and A. Meheust. 2010. "Prebiotic Effects: Metabolic and Health Benefits." *British Journal of Nutrition* 104, no. S2, pp. S1–63. doi:10.1017/s0007114510003363

Rosenfeldt, F.L., S.J. Haas, H. Krum, A. Hadj, K. Ng, J.Y. Leong, and G.F. Watts. 2007. "Coenzyme 010 in the Treatment of Hypertension: A Meta-Analysis of the Clinical Trials." *Journal of Human Hypertension*, pp. 297–306. doi:10.1038/sj.jhh.1002138

Ryan, A.S., J.D. Astwood, S. Gautier, C.N. Kuratko, E.B. Nelson, and N. Salem. 2010. "Effects of Long-Chain Polyunsaturated Fatty Acid Supplementation on Neurodevelopment in Childhood: A Review of Human Studies." *Prostaglandins Leukotrienes and Essential Fatty Acids (PLEFA)* 82, no. 4–6, pp. 305–14. doi:10.1016/j.plefa.2010.02.007

Schuchardt, J.P., M. Huss, M. Stauss-Grabo, and A. Hahn. 2010. "Significance of Long-Chain Polyunsaturated Fatty Acids (PUFAs) for the Development and Behaviour of Children." *European Journal of Pediatrics* 169, no. 2, pp. 149–64. doi:10.1007/s00431-009-1035-8

Schuchardt, J.P., I. Schneider, H. Meyer, J. Neubronner, C. von Schacky, and A. Hahn. 2011. "Incorporation of EPA and DHA into Plasma Phospholipids in Response to Different Omega-3 Fatty Acid Formulations--A Comparative Bioavailability Study of Fish Oil vs. Krill Oil." *Lipids in Health and Diseases* 10, no. 1, p. 145. doi:10.1186/1476-511x-10-145

Scroggie, D.A., A. Albright, and M.D. Harris. 2003. "The Effect of Glucosamine-Chondroitin Supplementation on Glycosylated Hemoglobin Levels in Patients with Type 2 Diabetes Mellitus: A Placebo-Controlled, Double-Blinded, Randomized Clinical Trial." *Archives of Internal Medicine* 163, no. 13, pp. 1587–90. doi:10.1001/archinte.163.13.1587

Serhan, C.N., N. Chiang, J. Dalli, and B.D. Levy. 2014. "Lipid Mediators in the Resolution of Inflammation." *Cold Spring Harbor Perspectives in Biology* 7, no. 2: a016311. doi:10.1101/cshperspect.a016311

Setnikar, L., C. Giacchetti, and G. Zanolo. 1986. "Pharmacokinetics of Glucosamine in the Dog and in Man." *Arzneimittelforschung* 36, no. 4, pp. 729–35.

Setnikar, L., R. Palumbo, S. Canali, and G. Zanolo. 1993. "Pharmacokinetics of Glucosamine in Man." *Arzneimittelforschung* 43, no. 10, pp. 1109–13.

Shanahan, F. 2002. "Probiotics and Inflammatory Bowel Disease: From Fads and Fantasy to Facts and Future." *British Journal of Nutrition* 88, no. S1, pp. S5–S9. doi:10.1079/bjn2002624

Sinatra, S.T. 2009. "Metabolic Cardiology: An Integrative Strategy in the Treatment of Congestive Heart Failure." *Alternative Therapies in Health and Medicine* 15, no. 3, pp. 44–52.

Smit, E.N., F.A.J. Muskiet, and E. Rudy Boersma. 2004. "The Possible Role of Essential Fatty Acids in the Pathophysiology of Malnutrition: A Review." *Prostaglandins Leukotrienes and Essential Fatty Acids* 71, no. 4, pp. 241–50. doi:10.1016/j.plefa.2004.03.019

Tannis, A.J., J. Barban, and J.A. Conquer. 2004. "Effect of Glucosamine Supplementation on Fasting and Non-Fasting Plasma Glucose and Serum Insulin Concentrations in Healthy Individuals." *Osteoarthritis and Cartilage* 12, no. 6, pp. 506–11. doi:10.1016/j.joca.2004.03.001

Thie, N.M., N.G. Prasad, and P.W. Major. 2001. "Evaluation of Glucosamine Sulfate Compared to Ibuprofen for the Treatment of Temporomandibular Joint Osteoarthritis: A Randomized Double Blind Controlled 3 Month Clinical Trial." *Journal of Rheumatology* 28, no. 6, pp. 1347–55.

Thien, F.C.K., R.K. Woods, and M.J. Abramson. 2002. "Dietary Marine Fatty Acids (Fish Oil) for Asthma in Adults and Children." *Cochrane Database Systematic Reviews* 3: CD001283. doi:10.1002/14651858.CD001283

Uebelhart, D., E.J. Thonar, P.D. Delmas, A. Chantraine, and E. Vignon. 1998. "Effects of Oral Chondroitin Sulfate on the Progression of Knee Osteoarthritis: A Pilot Study." *Osteoarthritis and Cartilage* 6 Suppl A, pp. 39–46. doi:10.1016/s1063-4584(98)80011-3

Uebelhart, D., M. Malaise, R. Marcolongo, F. de Vathaire, M. Piperno, E. Mailleux, A. Fioravanti, L. Matoso, and E. Vignon. 2004. "Intermittent Treatment of Knee Osteoarthritis with Oral Chondroitin Sulfate: a One-Year, Randomized, Double-Blind, Multicenter Study Versus Placebo." *Osteoarthritis and Cartilage* 12, no. 4, pp. 269–76. doi:10.1016/j.joca.2004.01.004

Uitterlinden, E.J., H. Jahr, J.L. Koevoet, Y.M. Jenniskens, S.M. Bierma-Zeinstra, J. Degroot, J.A. Verhaar, H. Weinans, and G.J. van Osch. 2006. "Glucosamine Decreases Expression of Anabolic and Catabolic Genes in Human Osteoarthritic Cartilage Explants." *Osteoarthritis and Cartilage* 14, no. 3, pp. 250–57. doi:10.1016/j.joca.2005.10.001

USDA. 2010. *Dietary Guidelines for Americans 2010.* Washington, DC: U.S. Government Printing Office.

USDA. 2012. *Nutrient Intakes from Food: Mean Amounts Consumed per Individual, by Gender and Age, What We Eat in America, NHANES 2009–2010.* Washington, DC: USDA.

Vangsness, C.T., Jr., W. Spiker, and J. Erickson. 2009. "A Review of Evidence-Based Medicine for Glucosamine and Chondroitin Sulfate use in Knee Osteoarthritis." *Arthroscopy* 25, no. 1, pp. 86–94. doi:10.1016/j.arthro.2008.07.020

Wang, C., and M. Chung. 2004. Effects of Omega-3 Fatty Acids on Cardiovascular Disease. Rockville, MD: Agency for Healthcare Research and Quality.

Wei, Y.H., S.B. Wu, Y.S. Ma, and H.C. Lee. 2009. "Respiratory Function Decline and DNA Mutation in Mitochondria, Oxidative Stress and Altered Gene Expression during Aging." *Chang Gung Medical Journal* 32, no. 2, pp. 113–32.

Wildi, L.M., J.P. Raynauld, J. Martel-Pelletier, A. Beaulieu, L. Bessette, F. Morin, F. Abram, M. Dorais, and J.P. Pelletier. 2011. "Chondroitin Sulphate Reduces both Cartilage Volume Loss and Bone Marrow Lesions in Knee Osteoarthritis Patients Starting as Early as 6 Months After Initiation of Therapy: A Randomised, Double-Blind, Placebo-Controlled Pilot Study Using MRI." *Annuals of Rheumatic Diseases* 70, no. 6, pp. 982–89. doi:10.1136/ard.2010.140848

Wyman, M., M. Leonard, and T. Morledge. 2010. "Coenzyme 010: A Therapy for Hypertension and Statin-Induced Myalgia?" *Cleveland Journal of Clinical Medicine* 77, no. 7, pp. 435–42. doi:10.3949/ccjm.77a.09078

Young, J.M., C.M. Florkowski, S.L. Molyneux, R.G. McEwan, C.M. Frampton, M.G. Nicholls, R.S. Scott, and P.M. George. 2012. "A Randomized, Double-Blind, Placebo-Controlled Crossover Study of Coenzyme Q10 Therapy in Hypertensive Patients with the Metabolic Syndrome." *American Journal of Hypertension* 25, no. 2, pp. 261–70. doi:10.1038/ajh.2011.209

Ziai, S.A., B. Larijani, S. Akhoondzadeh, H. Fakhrzadeh, A. Dastpak, F. Bandarian, A. Rezai, H.N. Badi, and T. Emami. 2005. "Psyllium Decreased Serum Glucose and Glycosylated Hemoglobin Significantly in Diabetic Outpatients." *Journal of Ethnopharmacology* 102, no. 2, pp. 202–7. doi:10.1016/j.jep.2005.06.042

CHAPTER 4

Survey of the 20 Most Common Dietary Supplements—Herbs and Botanicals

Overview

This chapter reviews five of the most popular herbal dietary supplements. These five consist of green tea, garlic, cranberry, echinacea, and ginseng. The background, traditional use, and clinical evidence exploring the properties and potential health benefits of each are discussed. The safety of each supplement are also discussed.

Introduction

A botanical, by definition, is a plant or part of a plant valued for its medicinal or therapeutic properties. Products made from botanicals are called herbal products, botanical products, phytomedicines, or nutraceuticals. These may include teas in addition to other product forms. Most herbal products differ from other dietary supplements in that they do not usually contain essential nutrients but contain, instead, phyto-chemicals believed to have some beneficial drug-like effect on the body or some unique antioxidant property. In addition, most herbal products sold as dietary supplements are known for their "traditional use." The traditional use of a product refers to the presence and use of a botanical within cultural medicine systems. Examples include traditional Chinese Medicine and Ayurvedic Medicine. Traditional use can refer to a historic use no longer in practice or to those used medicinally even today.

With herbal products, benefits can be claimed for any known area of health. This is due to the tremendous variety of phytochemicals they contain. This variety of chemicals also poses risks, in that oftentimes the chemicals in herbal products interact with each other. Some may act synergistically together, while others may counteract each other. Some benefits may be additive for a specific effect whereas others may be entirely unrelated to one another. I tell people taking a herbal product for a specific benefit is like trying to calm a headache by opening up a medicine cabinet full of over the counter medicines, and taking one pill from each bottle because you know one of them contains an aspirin.

This chapter reviews five of the most popular consumer herbal products in the market today. The benefits they offer range from preventing urinary tract infections (UTIs) to supporting heart health and several things in-between. I should mention that the five herbal supplements we discuss in this chapter constitute a very small selection of the large herbal product category. There is a far greater variety of herbal products on the market than any other dietary supplement category.

Green Tea

Background

According to legend, the first cup of tea was brewed by a Chinese emperor some 4,000 years ago. Since then, green tea has had a place in traditional Chinese medicine as a remedy for many things including headaches, body aches and pains, digestion, depression, immunity, low energy, and aging.

All teas (i.e., green, black, and oolong) are derived from the same plant, *Camellia sinensis*. *C. sinensis* is a member of the Theaceae family. The difference between the types of teas is in how the leaves are prepared. Green tea, unlike black and oolong, is not fermented, so the active constituents remain unoxidized. Not only are green tea leaves not fermented they are steamed, which inactivates the enzymes responsible for oxidation, thus preserving the active *compounds* in their original form.

Tea is one of the most widely consumed beverages in the world, second only to water. A great deal of research has been done to understand the chemical composition and health effects of green tea. About 30 to 40 percent of the compounds in an extract of green tea leaves are polyphenols. One class of polyphenol, in particular called flavanols, play an important role in the health benefits of green tea. These flavanols are comprised mostly of compounds called catechins namely, epigallocatechin-3-gallate (EGCG), epi-gallocatechin (EGC), epicatechin gallate (ECG), and epicatechin (EC). EGCG is present in the highest concentration and is perhaps the most potent.

Because of the long history of traditional use (i.e., millennia), green tea has been recommended for many ailments from cavities to cancer and everything in between. The most researched properties of green tea center on its antioxidant activity, its ability to promote weight loss, and its anticancer properties. Most recently, green tea has been examined for its prebiotic properties as well.

Green tea's antioxidant potential is directly related to the combination of aromatic rings and hydroxyl groups of the polyphenols it contains. The structure of these molecules enables the binding and neutralization of free radicals by the hydroxyl groups. The oxygen radical absorbance capacity assay is commonly utilized to measure the antioxidant capacity of plant-based antioxidants. Units are expressed as trolox equivalents, and green tea provides ~1,300 µmol of trolox equivalents per gram of dried tea leaves (Forester 2011).

Green tea's connection to weight loss stems from its caffeine content as well as its interaction with an enzyme called catechol-O-methyltransferase (COMT). COMT deactivates catecholamines such as dopamine, epinephrine, and norepinephrine. Green tea polyphenols are a substrate for this enzyme and can reduce its activity leading to increased serum levels of catecholamines in the body (Dulloo et al. 2000; Lu, Meng, and Yang 2003). Both norepinephrine and epinephrine are lipolytic, meaning they stimulate the breakdown and release of stored fat from fat cells. As a COMT inhibitor, green tea polyphenols have the potential to increase the level and duration of activity of these lipolytic catecholamines.

The mechanistic role of green tea in cancer metabolism is multifaceted. EGCG and ECG are potent antioxidants and may protect cells from DNA damage caused by reactive oxygen species. Green tea polyphenols stimulate detoxification systems; they can induce phase I and phase II metabolic enzymes that increase the degradation of carcinogens; they inhibit biochemical markers of tumor initiation and promotion, including lowering the rate of cell replication and thus the growth and development of neoplasms; and they prevent mutagenicity and genotoxicity (Brown 1999).

Rationale for Supplementation

Most consumers of green tea supplements take them because they believe that there are overall health benefits to taking it. This makes sense considering the beneficial properties of polyphenols discussed previously. Besides general wellness, many consumers take green tea or products with green tea ingredients for specific purposes, particularly, weight loss and cancer. More recently, polyphenols such as those found in green tea have been studied for their ability to enhance beneficial gut flora (Cardona et al. 2013; Dueñas et al. 2015).

The evidence for the efficacy of green tea extract in weight loss is mixed. A recent double blind study showed that EGCG at a daily dose of ~860 mg for 12 weeks produced significant weight loss, reduced waist circumference, and improved cholesterol profile without side effects in women with central obesity (Chen et al. 2015). This is in contrast to a review of 15 different placebo-controlled studies involving 1,945 subjects that was unable to demonstrate a consistent statistically significant effect on weight loss after 12 to 13 weeks of green tea supplementation (Jurgens et al. 2012). Looking closely at the data, however, reveals that in studies that failed to show statistical significance, there are individuals who did have clinically relevant results. This could have happened due to at least three reasons. First, green tea extracts differ in the levels of not only polyphenols but also caffeine. Green tea affects weight loss in part because of its caffeine content. Caffeine is able to increase levels of catecholamines such as norepinephrine in the body, which is synergistic with green tea's ability to inhibit COMT. If the studies in question used green tea extracts that differed in their polyphenol and caffeine content, this could affect the results. Second, there appears to be some genetic variability in the activity on COMT (Inoue-Choi et al. 2010; Miller et al. 2012). Because the mechanism of green tea involves COMT, any variation in its activity from subject to subject could explain why some individuals experienced meaningful weight loss and others did not. Finally, there is the issue of absorption. There is evidence that tea catechins such as EGCG are very poorly absorbed, perhaps less than 2 percent of what is ingested (Warden et al. 2001). Factors such as taking it on an empty stomach or with a meal affect absorption; with absorption *increasing* when taken on an empty stomach. At the same time, fish oil has been shown to increase the bioavailability of EGCG in mice (Giunta et al. 2010). This too could have affected the outcome in many studies that looked at green tea supplementation and weight loss.

In addition to weight loss, people sometimes look to green tea extract for its anticancer properties. As discussed previously, green tea polyphenols such as EGCG and ECG show mechanistic involvement in many processes relating to cancer growth and development. In animal studies, green tea polyphenols have also been shown to inhibit tumor cell proliferation and induce apoptosis of cancer cells (Lambert and Yang 2003). In addition, tea polyphenols may protect against skin damage caused by UV radiation. Furthermore, green tea has been shown to stimulate detoxification systems, specifically selective induction or modification of glutathione S-transferase and quinone reductase, that may help protect against tumor development (National Cancer Institute 2010; Steele et al. 2000).

In vitro animal and epidemiological studies are very promising showing anticancer effects against many types of cancer. Human clinical trials, however, have not shown the same efficacy. In a double-blind placebo-controlled study, involving men with high-grade prostatic intraepithelial neoplasia, which is thought to be a precursor of prostate cancer, 1 in 30 subjects had detectable prostate cancer following one year of supplementation compared to 9 in 30 men in the placebo group (Bettuzzi et al. 2006). This is contrasted by two uncontrolled studies that were unable to show significant activity against cancer in patients with existing prostate carcinoma (Choan et al. 2005; Jatoi et al. 2003). At best, the evidence supporting the use of green tea extract for cancer prevention is inconclusive.

The broadest benefits of green tea extract could come from its ability to interact with microbial populations in the gut. Interest in the microbiome has grown precipitously within the last decade. The microbiome consists of all the genes of living organisms that live on the surface of the body.

The gastrointestinal tract presents a large surface area with favorable conditions for microbes, particularly bacteria. The large majority of bacteria found in the gut play an important role in human health. There are no transporters for polyphenols to be absorbed from the gut. They must cross the gut barrier through passive diffusion, and it is known that only a very small percentage (<2 percent) of the polyphenols are absorbed intact. Unabsorbed polyphenols travel through the gastrointestinal tracts and end up in the large bowel where they are metabolized by bacteria. In fact, many of the beneficial effects attributed to polyphenols may be due to phenolic metabolites produced by gut bacteria that are more bioavailable (Dueñas et al. 2015). Additionally, beneficial gut bacteria increase in number after green tea consumption (Jin et al. 2012).

Safety

Consumption of green tea is considered safe as attested by the thousands of years of its use. Green tea extracts, however, present the body with much higher doses of polyphenols and other substances than can be achieved by drinking tea. There have been reports of cases of elevated liver enzymes following green tea extract supplementation. It is unknown, however, if these events were caused by the green tea or by the presence of impurities or adulterants in some commercial products. Green extract supplements can be considered safe when taken as directed. As always, it is good to consult your physician or health care provider before taking any nutraceutical-type product.

Garlic

Background

Garlic is a fragrant culinary herb from the genus and species *Allium sativum* which has been traditionally used worldwide for centuries. Garlic is made up of more than 200 chemicals including the sulfur compounds (allicin, alliin, and agoene); volatile oils; enzymes (allinase, peroxidase, and miracynase); carbohydrates (sucrose and glucose); minerals; amino acids such as cysteine, glutamine, isoleucine, and methionine; bioflavonoids such as quercetin and cyanidin; and vitamins A, C, E, B1, B2, niacin, and beta-carotene.

The beneficial properties of garlic are most commonly tied to their organosulfur compounds. Whole garlic bulbs contain alliin (S-allylcysteine (SAC) sulfoxide), gamma-glutamyl-S-allylcysteine (GSAC), S-methyl-cysteine sulfoxide (methiin), S-trans-1-propenylcysteine sulfoxide, and S-2-carboxypropylglutathione and SAC. Cutting, crushing, or grinding garlic releases the enzyme alliinase, which very quickly converts alliin to allicin. Allicin is responsible for the pungent odor and taste of garlic. Allicin is easily transformed into oil-soluble polysulfides, namely, diallyl disulfide, diallyl sulfide, diallyl trisulfide (DATS), and diallyl tetrasulfide. Because of allicin's instability, it is unlikely that it is responsible for the biological activity of garlic. An active component of garlic, Ajoene (4, 5, 9-trithiadodeca-1, 6, 11-triene-9-oxide) is generated via allicin S-thiolation and 2-propenesulfenic acid addition. Other active compounds, SAC and S-allylmercaptocysteine (SAMC) are water-soluble compounds formed during aqueous garlic extraction.

Metabolism of garlic is not well understood. Some studies have focused on compounds measured in expired air; however, this is not a reliable representation of blood levels from oral supplementation. There is some data available, however, regarding the metabolism of SAC in animals and humans. Animal studies have found SAC levels in the blood correlate with administered SAC doses, and urine levels of N-acetyl-S-allylcysteine following oral administration of SAC indicate that SAC can be transformed by N-acetyltransferase (Jandke and Spiteller 1987; Nagae et al. 1994). SAC has also been reported in human blood with ingestion of aged garlic extract (AGE), which has high levels of SAC (Steiner and Li 2001).

Garlic is available in several different forms. The most crude form is the sliced fresh herb, providing ~4 g from one clove. Garlic powder is produced from crushed garlic cloves, and is most commonly provided in 200 to 300 mg dosages with a recommended intake of three times a day. The powder contains alliin and a small amount of oil-soluble sulfur compounds. It does not contain any allicin. Garlic extracts are generated by soaking sliced garlic cloves in an extraction solution for a specified period of time and then concentrating the solution. The most common garlic extract product is the AGE, Kyolic. Kyolic is an ethanol extraction product. The extraction and aging process of this product allows the odorous compounds of the garlic to naturally transform into stable odorless compounds. Kyolic is most commonly sold in dosages of 300 to 800 mg dosages, also recommended to be taken three times daily. This product contains SAC, SAMC, and allyl sulfides.

Rationale for Supplementation

Garlic has been one of the top selling dietary supplements in the United States for many years. In 2000, garlic was ranked third in retail sales in the mass market, generating revenues of greater than $61 million (Blumenthal 2001). Garlic is most commonly used as a supplement for its cardiovascular benefits including lipid-lowering, antihypertensive, antithrombotic effects. The lipid-lowering benefits of garlic are attributed to several mechanisms. Garlic supplementation inhibits cholesterol biosynthesis at the level of beta-hydroxy-beta-methylglutaryl-CoA (HMG-CoA) reductase (Gebhardt 1993; Gebhardt, Beck, and Wagner 1994; Yeh and Yeh 1994; Yeh et al. 1995). Garlic also inhibits cholesterol biosynthesis by enhancing the palmitate-induced inhibition of cholesterol biosynthesis and targeting squalene monooxygenase, the enzyme that catalyzes the downstream pathway in cholesterol synthesis (Gebhardt 1995; Gupta and Porter 2001). Some forms of garlic also contain steroid saponins, which interfere with the absorption of total and low-density lipoprotein (LDL) cholesterol (Matsuura 2001). Antihypertensive benefits of garlic are most likely a result of the gamma-glutamylcysteine and fructan content of the herb. Gamma-glutamylcysteine inhibits angiotensin-converting enzyme, which leads to an inhibition of angiotensin II (Lawson 1998; Sendl et al. 1992). Angiotensin II is a hormone responsible for increasing vasoconstriction; therefore, its inhibition results in vasodilation. Fructans inhibit adenosine deaminase, which results in an increase in adenosine, which is responsible for blood vessel dilation (Koch et al. 1992; Lawson 1998). Multiple possible mechanisms are believed responsible for the antithrombotic effects of garlic. Garlic supplementation inhibits platelet aggregation and stimulates fibrinolysis. These benefits have been attributed to allicin and thiosulfinates at low doses and to cycloalliin at high doses (Lawson 1998; Reuter, Koch, and Lawson 1996). Garlic has also been found to inhibit the synthesis of prostaglandins and thromboxanes through the inhibition of lipoxygenase and cyclooxygenase pathways of the arachidonic acid cascade (Rahman and Billington 2000; Reuter, Koch, and Lawson 1996). These compounds are associated with platelet aggregation. The Ajoene found in garlic also affects fibrinogen-induced human platelet aggregation and inhibits binding of fibrinogen to adenosine diphosphate-stimulated platelets (Reuter, Koch, and Lawson 1996). Several human clinical studies have reported positive benefits of garlic supplementation for cardiovascular health benefits, and a review by the Agency for Healthcare Research and Quality concluded that garlic preparations may have small, positive, short-term effects on lipids and promising antithrombotic effects (Auer et al. 1990; Grunwald et al. 1992; Holzgartner, Schmidt, and Kuhn 1992; Jain et al. 1993; Lau, Lam, and Wang-Cheng 1987; Mader 1990; Steiner and Lin 1994; Steiner et al. 1996; Vorberg and Schneider 1990; Yeh et al. 1995).

Garlic is also supplemented to support immune function. The immunomodulatory benefits of garlic are believed to be attributed to the protein fraction of the herb (Lau, Yamasaki, and Grindley 1991). These fractions have been shown to inhibit activation of nuclear factor kappa B (NF-κB) in T-cells and increase phagocytosis, natural killer (NK) cell activity, antibody titers, and lymphocyte counts (Brosch and Platt 1993; Geng, Rong, and Lau 1997; Kandil et al. 1988; Lawson 1998). A human clinical study providing 2.56 g/day of AGE reported a significant reduction in the severity of cold and flu symptoms as well as improved proliferation of gamma–delta T-cells and NK cells (Nantz et al. 2012).

Antimicrobial effects against *Helicobacter pylori*, the bacteria implicated in some stomach cancers and ulcers, have led some consumers to reach for garlic to support gastric health. Garlic extracts have inhibited *H. pylori* in vitro, but when taken orally in human clinical studies, garlic has not been able to produce significant benefits for gastric health (Adetumbi and Lau 1983; Cavallito, Buck, and Suter 1944; Sivam 2001; Sivam et al. 1997).

The water-soluble compounds in garlic extracts, SAC and SAMC, have high antioxidant potential (Corzo-Martinez, Corzo, and Villamiel

2007). AGE garlic sources, which are higher in these compounds have a higher antioxidant capacity compared with fresh garlic extracts (Harauma and Moriguchi 2006). Some antioxidant action has also been reported for allicin and thiosulfinates. Garlic supplementation increases the activity of endogenous enzymes including glutathione peroxidase and catalase. It has also been shown to decrease the concentration of lipid peroxides in the blood (Geng and Lau 1997; Han, Liu, and Wang 1992; Ide and Lau 1999; Steiner and Lin 1994).

Safety

Garlic supplementation is safe when consumed at recommended dosages, and long-term use, up to seven years, has not resulted in any serious complications. Moreover, long-term supplementation is generally advised to allow for the cardiovascular benefits of garlic to take effect (Koscielny et al. 1999). The most commonly reported adverse events with garlic supplementation is the odor permeating the breath and skin, with more reports associated with raw garlic than with the cooked form (Blumenthal et al. 1998). Other reported adverse events include changes to the intestinal flora, allergic reactions, postoperative bleeding, spontaneous spinal epidural hematoma, platelet dysfunction, and increased clotting time; however, these events are rare (Brinckmann and Wollschlaeger 2003).

Garlic is contraindicated for use with three prescription drugs. Isoniazid (INH, Nydrazid), Non-Nucleoside Reverse Transcriptase Inhibitors, and saquinavir (Fortovase, Invirase) should be avoided with garlic supplementation (Dhamija, Malhotra, and Pandhi 2006; Piscitelli et al. 2002).

Cranberry

Background

American Cranberry (*Vaccinium macrocarpon* Ait.) is an evergreen shrub native to North America. It is indigenous to the eastern half of the United States. It can also be found in western Canada and down the western coast through California. Cranberry was used by Native Americans for medicinal purposes.

Today cranberry is cultivated primarily in Wisconsin, Massachusetts, New Jersey, Oregon, and Washington, and throughout Canada. Outside of North America, American Cranberry is cultivated in parts of Europe and Chile. Cranberries can be made into juices and sauces. It can be dried and used in breakfast cereals, snack bars, cheeses, and chocolate and other snack foods.

The health-promoting properties of cranberry are attributed to their high polyphenol content, which serve as a natural plant defense system against microbes. These polyphenols have been shown in vitro to have antibacterial, antiviral, antimutagenic, anticarcinogenic, antitumorigenic, antiangiogenic, anti-inflammatory, and antioxidant properties (Blumberg et al. 2013). Perhaps the most common health benefit attributed to cranberries is protection from UTIs.

The most studied cranberry polyphenol is a group of flavanols called A-type procyanidins (PACs). PACs can be found as A-type or B-type. The difference between A- and B-type PACs is important because their unique structures give them different biological properties. The A-type PACs exhibit significantly greater inhibition of *Escherichia coli* bacteria in cells that line the urinary tract than the B-type PACs. Adhesion of *E. coli* to cells lining the urinary tract is believed to be the first step in the development of a UTI. The level of A-type PACs can be used as a measure of quality of cranberry extracts. Other foods, such as apple, grape, and chocolate, contain high amounts of PACs, but only a few (plums, peanuts, avocados, cinnamon) contain A-type PACs, and none of these at the level found in cranberries.

In addition to PACs, cranberries are rich in anthocyanins, phenolic acids, and terpenes. Anthocyanins, which increase as the fruit ripens, are responsible for the deep red color of cranberries. There are many different structural varieties of anthocyanins in cranberries, and this is believed to influence the bioavailability and health effects of cranberries. Cranberry also contains phenolic acids, including hydroxybenzoic and hydroxycinnamic acids, hydroxybenzoic acid being the most abundant. A unique terpene known as ursolic acid is also present in cranberry. Interestingly, ursolic acid is a constituent of many medicinal remedies (Ikeda, Murakami, and Ohigashi 2008). Ursolic acid has strong anti-inflammatory properties. In addition to cranberry, ursolic acid can be found in apple skins, guavas, olives, and several herbs.

Cranberry obviously contains a large number of biologically active compounds including many not included in this discussion (e.g., quercetin). For our purposes, however, we have touched on those most believed to be responsible for cranberry's unique health-promoting properties.

Unfortunately, you cannot eat cranberries straight off the vine. Many of the phytochemicals we mentioned also give cranberry a very tart and astringent taste. Cranberry is mainly consumed as a juice blended with other sweet fruit juices to mask the astringent taste. The steps involved in the processing of cranberries into juice removes a good deal of the polyphenols and is damaging to many of the beneficial compounds. It is known that meaningful amounts of PACs are actually bound to the skin and that these PACs are made bioavailable in the digestive tract. Creating juice removes the skin and reduces the level of PACs. Some polyphenols are also sensitive to the higher temperatures used to pasteurize the juice and can be destroyed. Finally, oxidation (that occurs during processing) is also a significant reason why cranberry juice does not have the same levels of polyphenols as the raw fruit. Despite the loss of potency during processing, cranberry juice can still provide meaningful levels of polyphenols and the associated health benefits, if consumed regularly.

Rationale for Supplementation

Urinary Tract Infections

UTIs are the second most common type of infection. Over 8 million people seek medical care for UTIs each year (Schappert and Rechtsteiner 2008). UTIs are more common in women than men. A woman's urethra is shorter than a man's and allows bacteria to more easily reach the bladder. In addition, a woman's urethral opening is closer to sources of pathogenic bacteria such as the anus. These factors increase a woman's lifetime risk of getting a UTI to greater than 50 percent. UTIs in men are not as common as in women but can be just as serious when they occur.

UTIs are traditionally treated with antibiotics. The risk of developing antibiotic resistance and damaging the microbiome justify seeking alternative means to treat and prevent UTIs. The most common dietary supplement used for UTIs is cranberry. Most cranberry supplements are powders made by dehydrating the juice.

There are three possible mechanisms by which cranberries help to prevent UTIs (Hisano et al. 2012). First, in vitro studies have shown that cranberry is able to prevent adhesion of pathogenic bacteria to the cells lining the urethra and bladder. *E. coli* is the primary bacteria responsible for UTIs. The strains of *E. coli* associated with UTIs have protein tendrils called "fimbriae" on their surface that allow them to bind to cells of the urinary tract. This is believed to be the first step leading to infection. If the bacteria cannot adhere to the cells, they cannot become established and cause infection. Second, in vitro studies show that cranberry is able to alter the morphology of bacteria. Cranberry appears to reduce the number of the fimbriae extending from the surface of the bacteria and thereby reduce their ability to adhere. Again, if the bacteria are unable to bind to cells because of dysfunctional or missing fimbriae they cannot become established and cause infection. Finally, and this is speculation on the author's part, it is possible that through a prebiotic effect, cranberry polyphenols may improve the number of beneficial bacteria, thereby reducing the number of pathogenic bacteria in the large bowel, lowering the risk of cross contaminating the urethra.

Cranberry has been studied in a number of different groups who are susceptible to recurrent UTIs, among them, women who are pregnant, children, men, and individuals with neurogenic bladder dysfunction (Hisano et al. 2012). In 2008, the *Cochrane Database of Systematic Reviews* published a review of 10 randomized trials involving 1,049 patients. The review included studies using cranberry juice and cranberry supplement capsules. They concluded that there is some evidence that cranberry juice may decrease the number of symptomatic UTIs over a 12-month period, in particularly, and only, for women with recurrent UTIs (Jepson and Craig 2008). Despite this limited finding by *Cochrane Reviews*, clearly demonstrating that cranberry is effective at preventing the recurrence of UTIs has been difficult and very inconsistent.

There are a number of reasons why in vivo studies of cranberry and UTIs have not been consistently positive (Blumberg et al. 2013; Hisano et al. 2012). The minimum effective dose of cranberry extract for the prevention of UTIs is not currently known. In addition, the level of active polyphenols in cranberry beverages vary widely even from the same manufacturer. Most studies have used beverages containing 25 percent cranberry juice. Even when the percentage of juice is controlled for, the actual amount of active compounds in the juice is not standardized.

Another possible reason why outcomes from cranberry trials have been inconsistent is the high dropout rates reported. The number of subject dropouts in most studies varied considerably, ranging from 0 to as high as 55 percent. No consistent reason is evident for such high dropout rates, though in pediatric studies, the taste of cranberry juice is often cited as a reason for discontinuation.

Similar to the impact of dropout is noncompliance. Studies done with institutionalized subjects, such as the elderly, have seen a significant reduction in recurrent UTIs (Avorn et al. 1994), while several subsequent studies in the elderly living at home have not been consistently positive. Monitoring compliance is easier when subjects are living in a long-term care facility than in free-living conditions. When dropout rates are high or the level of compliance is unknown, accurate interpretation of the outcome data is significantly more difficult.

When looking at the evidence as a whole, it can be suggested that a daily dose of 240 to 300 mL of cranberry juice cocktail may prevent up to 50 percent of the recurrences of UTIs and can reduce the presence of pathogenic bacteria in the urine. Recommended doses of cranberry extract is 36 mg PACs per day divided into two or three daily doses.

Cardiovascular Health

Beyond urinary tract health, cranberry may provide benefits for cardiovascular health and act as a prebiotic. Several indexes of cardiovascular health may be improved by cranberry supplementation. Cardiovascular risk factors such as dyslipidemia, diabetes, hypertension, inflammation, oxidative stress, endothelial dysfunction, arterial stiffness, and platelet function have been examined with cranberry supplementation.

Cranberry consumption has been shown to lower LDL cholesterol and raise HDL cholesterol in animal models and in some human populations. Human trials showing improvements in blood lipid profiles include subjects with type 2 diabetes, and subjects with low HDL-C, and high triglycerides. Not all human trials, however, have demonstrated cranberry's ability to significantly improve blood lipids.

Animal studies have demonstrated that cranberry polyphenols lower blood glucose and improve insulin sensitivity in models of type 2 diabetes. Cranberry supplementation in human subjects, however, have yet to show a significant effect on glycemic control in patients with type 2 diabetes.

In vitro studies have shown that the cranberry polyphenols can inhibit angiotensin-converting enzyme, and thus have the potential to lower blood pressure. Cranberry extract prevented expected increase in blood pressure in hamsters fed a high-fat diet. Multiple trials using human subjects with existing cardiovascular disease and type 2 diabetes, however, failed to show blood pressure-lowering effects using cranberry juice. A study examining the effects of cranberry extract also showed no effect on blood pressure in subjects with untreated hypertension (Blumberg et al. 2013).

It is well established that cranberry polyphenols have antioxidant effects in vitro and in vivo in experimental models, and it seems plausible that these antioxidant properties might play a role in the cardiovascular benefits of cranberry supplementation. There is some evidence that consumption of cranberry juice or cranberry supplements improves blood markers of oxidative stress in healthy subjects and in patients with cardiovascular risk factors. For example, reduced levels of oxidized LDL cholesterol have been seen following cranberry supplementation. Nevertheless, most studies to date have failed to provide evidence for an actual decrease in markers of oxidative damage. In light of this, it is still uncertain what role cranberry's antioxidant properties might play in cardiovascular health.

Systemic inflammation is considered a risk factor for cardiovascular disease. Cranberry polyphenols are known to have anti-inflammatory properties. In vitro studies show that cranberry extract suppresses the activation of macrophages and T-cells exposed to proinflammatory stimuli. As is often the case with cranberry research, the data is encouraging yet inconsistent. C-reactive protein (CRP) is a serum marker of system inflammation. CRP has been shown to be reduced following cranberry polyphenol supplementation (Zhu et al. 2013). This data is in contrast to similar studies, which were unable to show a significant effect (Blumberg et al. 2013).

Finally, a recent eight-week double-blind placebo-controlled study was done using cranberry juice with a standardized polyphenol content (Novotny et al. 2015). Diet was also controlled. Subjects had not been diagnosed with cardiovascular disease. After eight-weeks, serum tri-glycerides were lower after consuming cranberry juice daily. Subjects with higher baseline triglyceride levels tended to show a greater improvement. Serum CRP was lower for subjects consuming cranberry than for subjects in the placebo group. Diastolic blood pressure was lower compared with the placebo group. Fasting blood sugar was lower in the cranberry group than in the placebo group and tended to improve more in those subjects with higher faster blood sugar levels at baseline.

Gut Health

Microbes in the digestive tract play a critical role in transforming dietary polyphenols such as those in cranberry into absorbable biologically active compounds (Marchesi et al. 2015). Less than 5 percent of dietary poly-phenols that reach the colon go unmetabolized by gut microbes (Clifford 2004). Khoo et al. conducted a randomized, double-blind, cross-over study comparing the effects of consuming a low sugar cranberry juice or placebo on fecal microbes and urine metabolites (Khoo et al. 2010). Levels of the beneficial bacteria bifidobacteria were significantly increased following cranberry juice supplementation for six weeks. This shows that dietary polyphenols such as those from cranberry modulate the human gut microbiota toward a more health-promoting profile by increasing the relative abundance of bifidobacteria.

Safety

Cranberries have been consumed as a food throughout recorded history and are generally recognized being safe as a food or food ingredient. Its safe use in whole form or even as juice does not necessarily imply, however, that highly concentrated cranberry extract is safe in all populations or at high levels of consumption. One possible area of concern is the risk of developing kidney stones. In a study of healthy volunteers consuming cranberry tablets for one week at the manufactures recommended dose, urinary oxalates were found to have increased significantly. While consumption of up to 4 L/day of cranberry juice has been shown to be nontoxic in healthy individuals, people with a history of stone formation may be at increased risk if they consume large amounts of cranberries or cranberry juice (Dugoua et al. 2008). In infants and young children, gastrointestinal distress, including diarrhea, has been reported when they consumed more than 3 L/day of cranberry juice.

Echinacea

Background

Echinacea is a hardy, perennial, medicinal plant belonging to the Aster family indigenous to the United States. Three species of the *Echinacea* genus, *E. purpurea* (L.) Moench, *E. pallida* (Nutt.) Nutt., and *E. augustifolia* DC, are most commonly used in dietary supplements to provide the health benefits of this plant. The most well-known health benefit for which echinacea is taken is immune support. Although research supports immune benefits from the other *Echinacea* species also, the *E. purpurea* species has been shown to have the strongest effect on the immune system (Bodinet, Willigmann, and Beuscher 1993). Echinacea supplements are prepared from the fresh above-ground parts, which are harvested when the plant is flowering, or the fresh or dried root. Echinacea is offered in several different preparations including juice, infusion, tincture, fluid extracts, and powdered extracts. In 1997, echinacea was the top-selling herbal supplement sold in all channels of trade in the United States bringing in $3.6 billion in total sales.

Echinacea plants contain many different constituents including alkamides, caffeic acid, caffeoyl derivatives, cichoric acid, cynarin, dodeca-2E,4E,8Z,10Z(E)-tetraenoic acid isobutylamides, dodecanoic acid derivatives, echinacoside, glycoconjugates, hydrophilic polysaccharides, N-isobutyldodeca-2E,4E,8Z,10Z-tetraenamide, pentadeca-(8Z,13Z)-dien-11-yn-2-one, polysaccharide, undeca-2-ene-8,10-diynoic acid isobutylamide, undecanoic acid derivatives, and unsaturated

N-alkylamide lipids. The amounts and concentrations of these constituents vary depending upon the species and the part of the echinacea plant used (Blumenthal 2003).

It appears the beneficial immune support effects of echinacea are tied to the multiple actions of various active compounds from the echinacea on multiple different components of the immune system. Echinacea has direct virucidal and bactericidal activities (Sharma et al. 2009, 2010). Alkamide-rich extracts of the herb are suggested to have anti-inflammatory benefits resulting in a reduction in 5-lipoxygenase and cyclooxygenase (Muller-Jakic et al. 1994). Echinacea has also been shown to reduce proinflammatory markers induced by pathogens including the secretion of interleukins IL-1, IL-6, and IL-8 and tumor necrosis factor-alpha (TNF-α). Glycoproteins and polysaccharides in the herb have been found to modulate certain immune cell functions including macrophages and NK cells (Bauer et al. 1989). Echinacea may also influence the activity of cytokines, reverse the excessive mucin secretion induced by viruses and modulate gene expression (Altamirano-Dimas et al. 2007; Burns et al. 2010; Hudson 2012; Sharma et al. 2010; Woelkart et al. 2005; Yin et al. 2010). It is believed that echinacea alkamides are absorbed into the blood and exert some of their effects through the endocannabinoid system (Chicca et al. 2009). As specific constituents of the herb may be tied to specific mechanisms, it is important to consider how preparations are prepared and if they are standardized to specific components of the plant when evaluating clinical research and using it to decide which products to purchase.

Echinacea has been used traditionally for centuries. The ethnobotanist M.R. Gilmore claims, "Echinacea seems to have been used as a remedy for more ailments than any other plant" (Gilmore 1911). It was one of the most commonly used medicines of Native Americans of the Great Plains. It is claimed they used it for toothache, mumps, sore throat, snakebite, coughs, burns, and pain relief (Foster 1991). Physicians in the 19th century prescribed echinacea for sepsis, mucous discharge, cancer, typhoid, fever, and skin sores (Felter and Lloyd 1898).

Rationale for Supplementation

Consumers turn to echinacea most often to help prevent and treat upper respiratory infections or colds (Barrett 2003). The common cold is the most common reason for which patients visit their primary care physicians. A large U.S. survey found that more than 70 percent of the population suffers from at least one cold per year (Fendrick 2003). As the common cold is caused by a virus, medical treatment options are limited, leading many patients to look for alternative treatment and prevention methods. A recent Cochrane review of the benefits of echinacea supplementation in preventing and treating the common cold found that the results of almost all of the prevention trials pointed in the direction of small preventive effects. In general, echinacea did not show significant reductions in illness occurrence (Karsch-Volk et al. 2014). The review does state that the great variety of forms of echinacea tested may have affected the ability to draw conclusions. Further, the report claims that some research does indicate that the effects of echinacea is likely due to several components that may have synergistic effects and that echinacea preparations standardized to specific compounds are more likely to produce benefits. Echinacea's benefits do appear to be most effective if supplementation is started as early as possible after symptoms are first noticed and is continued for 7 to 10 days. Prophylactic use of echinacea to decrease the odds of developing a cold has mixed clinical support (Barrett, Vohmann, and Calabrese 1999; Grimm and Muller 1999; Shah et al. 2007).

Because of its immune supporting properties, consumers also turn to echinacea for help in fighting other infections including UTIs, yeast infections, genital herpes. There is some research supporting oral and topical echinacea for the prevention of yeast infections (Coeugniet and Kuhnast 1986).

Although there is research supporting the use of echinacea for these conditions, dietary supplements are not allowed to be sold for the prevention or treatment of any disease or condition under Dietary Supplement Health and Education Act (DSHEA). Any echinacea products claiming to provide benefits beyond immune support would be in violation of the DSHEA regulations.

Safety

Echinacea supplementation is likely safe when taken orally at recommended dosages for short durations (up to 16 weeks) (Miller 1998). The most common reported adverse events with echinacea use are gastrointestinal upset, rash, and allergic reactions. There are moderate possibilities of interaction of echinacea with caffeine, cytochrome enzymes in the liver that metabolize many different drugs (e.g., acetaminophen, warfarin, lovastatin), and immunosuppressants (Bossaer and Odle 2012; Gorski et al. 2004; Stimpel et al. 1984; Yale and Glurich 2005).

Ginseng

Background

The term ginseng refers to a fleshy rooted plant belonging to several species of the genus *Panax*. The two most common species of ginseng are the Asian (*Panax ginseng*) and American (*Panax quinquefolius*) varieties. The active compounds used to characterize ginseng are triterpene glycosides called ginsenosides. Different species of ginseng can be distinguished by their ginsenoside content. The most commonly studied ginsenosides are Rb1, Rg1, Rg3, and Rd. Different parts of the plant may also include amino acids, alkaloids, phenols, proteins, polypeptides, and vitamins B1 and B2 (Blumenthal 2003). Standardized ginseng extracts are most commonly in the standardization range of 1 to 7 percent. Standardized doses usually range from 100 to 600 mg/day. Commercially, roots are graded according to source, age, part of the root used, and method of preparation.

Once ingested, ginsenosides are absorbed in the intestines after being metabolized in the stomach and by the bacteria in the digestive tract through a process called deglycosylation and esterification. Ginsenoside metabolism is initiated by the ginsenoside Rd pathway, and results in the production of Compound K (Cpd K). Once absorbed, ginsenosides are shown to enter into the brain rapidly, but their concentrations decline rapidly (Lee et al. 2009; Zhang et al. 2014).

The exact molecular mechanism by which ginseng imparts its health benefits is not entirely clear. Based on available in vitro and in vivo scientific evidence, it appears that the mechanisms may be linked to effects on the hypothalamus–pituitary–adrenal axis and the hypothalamus-pituitary–testis axis and the combined activities of anti-inflammatory, antioxidant, and immune cell enhancement effects (Kim et al. 2009;

Lee, Lee, and Kim 1998; Salvati et al. 1996; Scaglione et al. 1996; World Health Organization 1999). In the nervous system, ginseng appears to induce changes in corticosteroid, monoamine, and interleukin levels in the cortex and hippocampus regions of the brain (Rasheed et al. 2008). The major anti-inflammatory mechanisms are suppression of TNF-α NF-κB, prostaglandin E2 (PGE2), and cyclooxygenase-2 (COX-2) (Kang and Min 2012; Kim et al. 2013). There are also significant mechanisms related to modulation of NK cells and T-cells (Kang and Min 2012). Also, metabolites of ginsenosides such as Compound K and Ginsenoside Rp1 (G-Rp1) have been shown to have antioxidative and anti-inflammatory activities (Li and Zhong 2014; Shen et al. 2011).

Rationale for Supplementation

Ginseng is primarily used as an adaptogen, which is believed to increase resistance to stress and improve well-being. These benefits are attributed to ginseng's effects on the hypothalamic–pituitary–adrenal axis. This axis controls corticotropin and corticosteroid levels (Nocerino, Amato, and Izzo 2000). Antianxiety, antidepressant, and cognition-enhancing benefits of ginseng were originally recorded thousands of years ago by Shi-Zhen Li in *Ben Cao Gang Mu*, a premodern herbal book from the days of the Ming Dynasty (Ong et al. 2015). Despite reported traditional use of ginseng for adaptogenic benefits, human clinical research supporting these benefits is lacking. Animal data shows more promise, however (Wei et al. 2007).

Consumers also commonly use ginseng as an ergogenic aid, to improve endurance and athletic performance. Clinical support for ginseng's ergogenic properties is mixed. While some studies report an improvement in physical performance with ginseng supplementation (Cherdrungsi and Rungroeng 1995; Le Gal, Cathebras, and Struby 1996; Van Schepdael 1993), other clinical studies do not show significant benefits (Engels, Said, and Wirth 1996; Engels and Wirth 1997). A successful study providing 300 mg of ginseng per day for two months reported significant improvements in maximal oxygen uptake, resting heart rate, and leg strength compared with placebo (Cherdrungsi and Rungroeng 1995).

Ginseng supplementation is also commonly taken for cognitive function benefits. Clinical evidence demonstrates benefits of *P. ginseng* for abstract thinking, attention, mental arithmetic skills, and reaction times in adults (Kennedy et al. 2004; Reay, Kennedy, and Scholey 2005, 2006; Reay, Scholey, and Kennedy 2010; Sorensen and Sonne 1996). Significant benefits of a single 200 mg dose of *P. ginseng* were found in a clinical study involving 30 healthy young adults. Improvements in the Serial Sevens subtraction task and mental fatigue were also reported using a 10 minute test battery (Reay, Kennedy, and Scholey 2005).

Immune support is another common objective for ginseng supplementation. Clinical evidence supports the use of ginseng for this benefit. Proprietary ginseng extracts have been shown in clinical studies to have immunomodulatory effects in humans and reduce the frequency of influenza and the common cold (McElhaney et al. 2006; Predy et al. 2005; Scaglione et al. 1990; Scaglione et al. 1996). Supplementation with 200 mg/day of the ginseng extract G115 resulted in a significant reduction in frequency of influenza or common cold, as well as increased activity levels of NK cells, the immune system cells responsible for rapid immune responses (Scaglione et al. 1996).

Consumers also look to ginseng to support sexual health. Several human clinical studies support the use of ginseng for erectile dysfunction in men and sexual arousal in women (Amato, Izzo, and Nocerino 2000; Choi, Seong, and Rha 1995; Hong et al. 2002; Jang et al. 2008; Kim et al. 2009; Oh et al. 2010; Salvati et al. 1996). One study showed that 900 mg of Korean red ginseng taken three times daily resulted in a significant improvement in erectile function compared with those given a placebo (Hong et al. 2002). In menopausal women with reduced sexual drive, daily supplementation with 3 g/day of Korean red ginseng resulted in a significant improvement in the Female Sexual Function Index (Oh et al. 2010).

Safety

P. ginseng is generally well-tolerated, when taken orally at the recommend dosages for short time periods (up to six months). Potential hormone-like effects of ginseng creates some concern around long-term ginseng supplementation. Intake should be limited to time periods no longer than six months (Cho et al. 2004). Occasionally reported adverse effects included nausea, diarrhea, euphoria, insomnia, headaches, hypertension, hypotension, breast pain, and vaginal bleeding, which were mild and reversible (Kiefer and Pantuso 2003).

There are no known major drug interaction concerns for ginseng, but potential drug interaction risk exists for anticoagulant or antiplatelet drugs, antidiabetes drugs, cytochrome P450 substrates, estrogens, furosemide, immunosuppressants, insulin, and monoamine oxidase inhibitors (Becker et al. 1996; Caron et al. 2002; Gonzalez-Seijo, Ramos, and Lastra 1995; Gurley, Gardner, and Hubbard 2000; Jones and Runikis 1987; Lee et al. 1987, 2003; Mateo-Carrasco et al. 2012; Park et al. 1996; Shin et al. 2000; Smith, Lin, and Zheng 2001; Sotaniemi, Haapakoski, and Rautio 1995). Individuals should be cautious and consult their health care provider regarding these combinations.

References

Adetumbi, M.A., and B.H. Lau. 1983. "Allium Sativum (Garlic)—A Natural Antibiotic." *Medical Hypotheses* 12, no. 3, pp. 227–37. doi:10.1016/0306-9877(83)90040-3

Altamirano-Dimas, M., J.B. Hudson, D. Cochrane, C. Nelson, and J.T. Arnason. 2007. "Modulation of Immune Response Gene Expression by Echinacea Extracts: Results of a Gene Array Analysis." *Canadian Journal of Physiology Pharmacology* 85, no. 11, pp. 1091–98. doi:10.1139/Y07-110

Amato, M., A. Izzo, and E. Nocerino. 2000. "The Aphrodisiac and Adaptogenic Properties of Ginseng." *Fitoterapia* 71, pp. S1–S5. doi:10.1016/s0367-326x(00)00170-2

Auer, W., A. Eiber, E. Hertkorn, E. Hoehfeld, U. Koehrle, and A. Lorenz. 1990. "Hypertension and Hyperlipidemia: Garlic Helps in Mild Cases." *British Journal of Clinical Practice* 69, pp. 3–6.

Avorn, J., M. Monane, J.H. Gurwitz, R.J. Glynn, I. Choodnovskiy, and L.A. Lipsotz. 1994. "Reduction of Bacteriuria and Pyuria After Ingestion of Cranberry Juice." *JAMA: Journal of the American Medical Association* 271, no. 10, pp. 751–54. doi:10.1001/jama.271.10.751

Barrett, B. 2003. "Medicinal Properties of Echinacea." *Phytomedicine* 10, no. 1, pp. 66–86. doi:10.1078/094471103321648692

Barrett, B., M. Vohmann, and C. Calabrese. 1999. "Echinacea for Upper Respiratory Infection." *Journal of Family Practice* 48, no. 8, pp. 628–35.

Bauer, R., P. Remiger, K. Jurcic, and H. Wagner. 1989. "Effect of Extracts of Echinacea on Phagocytic Activity [Beeinflussung der Phagozytoseaktivitat Durch Echinacea-Extrakte]." *Zeitschrift Fur Phytherapie* 10, pp. 43–48.

Becker, B.N., J. Greene, J. Evanson, G. Chidsey, and W.J. Stone. 1996. "Ginseng-Induced Diuretic Resistance." *JAMA: The Journal of the American Medical Association* 276, no. 8, pp. 606–7. doi:10.1001/jama.1996.03540080028021

Bettuzzi, S., M. Brausi, F. Rizzi, G. Castagnetti, G. Peracchia, and A. Corti. 2006. "Chemoprevention of Human Prostate Cancer by Oral Administration of Green Tea Catechins in Volunteers with High-Grade Prostate Intraepithelial Neoplasia: A Preliminary Report from a One-Year Proof-of-Principle Study." *Cancer Research* 66, no. 2, pp. 1234–40. doi:10.1158/0008-5472.can-05-1145

Blumberg, J.B., T.A. Camesano, A. Cassidy, P. Kris-Etherton, A. Howell, C. Manach, L.M. Ostertag, H. Sies, A. Skulas-Ray, and J.A. Vita. 2013. "Cranberries and Their Bioactive Constituents in Human Health." *Advances in Nutrition* 4, no. 6, pp. 618–32. doi:10.3945/an.113.004473

Blumenthal, M. 2001. "Herb Sales Down 15% in Mainstream Market." *Herbal Gram* 51, p. 69.

Blumenthal, M. 2003. *The ABC Clinical Guide to Herbs*. Austin, TX: American Botanical Council.

Blumenthal, M. 2003. *The ABC Clinical Guide to Herbs*. New York, NY: Theime.

Blumenthal, M., W.R. Busse, A. Goldberg, J. Gruenwald, T. Hall, C.W. Riggins, and R. Rister, eds. 1988. *The Complete German Commission E Monographs: Therapeutic Guide to Herbal Medicines*. Translated by S. Klein and R. Rister. Boston, MA: Integrative Medicine Communication.

Bodinet, C., I. Willigmann, and N. Beuscher. 1993. "Host-Resistance Increasing Activity of Root Extracts from Echinacea Species." *Planta Medica* 59, no. Suppl, pp. a672–73. doi:10.1055/s-2006-959947

Bossaer, J.B., and B.L. Odle. 2012. "Probable Etoposide Interaction with Echinacea." *Journal of Dietary Supplements* 9, no. 2, p. 90–95. doi:10.3109/19390211.2012.682643

Brinckmann, J., and B. Wollschlaeger. 2003. "Garlic." In *The ABC Clinical Guide to Herbs*, eds. M. Blumenthal, T. Hall, A. Goldberg, T. Kunz, and K. Dinda. Austin, TX: American Botanical Council.

Brosch, T., and D. Platt. 1993. "About the Immunomodulatory Effect of Garlic (Allium Sativum)." *Med Welt* 44, pp. 309–13.

Brown, M.D. 1999. "Green Tea (Camellia Sinensis) Extract and Its Possible Role in the Prevention of Cancer." *Alternative Medicine Review* 4, no. 5, pp. 360–70.

Burns, J.J., L. Zhao, E.W. Taylor, and K. Spelman. 2010. "The Influence of Traditional Herbal Formulas on Cytokine Activity." *Toxicology* 278, no. 1, pp. 140–59. doi:10.1016/j.tox.2009.09.020

Cardona, F., C. Andrés-Lacueva, S. Tulipani, F.J. Tinahones, and M.I. Queipo-Ortuño. 2013. "Benefits of Polyphenols on Gut Microbiota and Implications in Human Health." *The Journal of Nutritional Biochemistry* 24, no. 8, pp. 1415–22. doi:10.1016/j.jnutbio.2013.05.001

Caron, M.F., A.L. Hotsko, S. Robertson, L. Mandybur, J. Kluger, and C.M. White. 2002. "Electrocardiographic and Hemodynamic Effects of Panax Ginseng." *The Annals Pharmacotherapy* 36, no. 5, pp. 758–63. doi:10.1345/1542-6270(2002)036<0758:eaheop>2.0.co;2

Cavallito, C., J. Buck, and C. Suter. 1944. "Allicin, the Antibacterial Principle of Allium Sativum. II. Determination of the Chemical Structure." *Journal of the American Chemical Society* 66, no. 11, pp. 1952–54. doi:10.1021/ja01239a049

Chen, I.J., C.Y. Liu, J.P. Chiu, and C.H. Hsu. 2015. "Therapeutic Effect of High-Dose Green Tea Extract on Weight Reduction: A Randomized, Double-Blind, Placebo-Controlled Clinical Trial." *Clinical Nutrition* S0261-5614(15)00134-X. doi:10.1016/j.clnu.2015.05.003

Cherdrungsi, P., and K. Rungroeng. 1995. "Effects of Standardized Ginseng Extract and Exercise Training on Aerobic and Anaerobic Exercise Capacities in Humans." *Korean Journal of Ginseng Research* 19, no. 2, pp. 93–100.

Chicca, A., S. Raduner, F. Pellati, T. Strompen, K.H. Altmann, R. Schoop, and J. Gertsch. 2009. "Synergistic Immunopharmacological Effects of N-alkylamides in Echinacea Purpurea Herbal Extracts." *International Immunopharmacology* 9, no. 7–8, pp. 850–58. doi:10.1016/j.intimp.2009.03.006

Cho, J., W. Park, S. Lee, W. Ahn, and Y. Lee. 2004. "Ginsenoside-Rb1 from Panax Ginseng C.A. Meyer Activates Estrogen Receptor-Alpha and -Beta, Independent of Ligand Binding." *The Journal of Clinical Endocrinology Metabolism* 89, no. 7, pp. 3510–15. doi:10.1210/jc.2003-031823

Choan, E., R. Segal, D. Jonker, S. Malone, N. Reaume, L. Eapen, and V. Gallant. 2005. "A Prospective Clinical Trial of Green Tea for Hormone Refractory Prostate Cancer: An Evaluation of the Complementary/Alternative Therapy Approach." *Urologic Oncology: Seminars and Original Investigations* 23, no. 2, 108–13. doi:10.1016/j.urolonc.2004.10.008

Choi, H., D. Seong, and K. Rha. 1995. "Clinical Efficacy of Korean Red Ginseng for Erectile Dysfunction." *International Journal of Impotence Research* 7, no. 3, pp. 181–86.

Clifford, M.N. 2004. "Diet-Derived Phenols in Plasma and Tissues and Their Implications for Health." *Planta Medica* 70, no. 12, pp. 1103–14. doi:10.1055/s-2004-835835

Coeugniet, E.G., and R. Kuhnast. 1986. "Recurrent Candidiasis: Adjuvant Immunotherapy with Different Formulations of Echinacin." *Therapiewoche* 36, pp. 3352–58.

Corzo-Martinez, M., N. Corzo, and M. Villamiel. 2007. "Biological Properties of Onions and Garlic." *Trends in Food Science & Technology* 18, no. 12, pp. 609–25. doi:10.1016/j.tifs.2007.07.011

Dhamija, P., S. Malhotra, and P. Pandhi. 2006. "Effect of Oral Administration of Crude Aqueous Extract of Garlic on Pharmacokinetic Parameters of Isoniazid and Rifampicin in Rabbits." *Pharmacology* 77, no. 2, pp. 100–104. doi:10.1159/000093285

Dueñas, M., I. Muñoz-González, C. Cueva, A. Jiménez-Girón, F. Sánchez-Patán, C. Santos-Buelga, M.V. Moreno-Arribas, and B. Bartolomé. 2015. "A Survey of Modulation of Gut Microbiota by Dietary Polyphenols." *Biomed Research International* 2015, pp. 1–15. doi:10.1155/2015/850902

Dugoua, J.J., D. Seely, D. Perri, E. Mills, and G. Koren. 2008. "Safety and Efficacy of Cranberry (Vaccinium Macrocarpon) During Pregnancy and Lactation." *The Canadian Journal of Clinical Pharmacology* 15, no. 1, pp. e80–86.

Dulloo, A.G., J. Seydoux, L. Girardier, P. Chantre, and J. Vandermander. 2000. "Green Tea and Thermogenesis: Interactions Between Catechin-Polyphenols, Caffeine and Sympathetic Activity." *International Journal of Obesity Relat Metab Disord* 24, no. 2, pp. 252–58. doi:10.1038/sj.ijo.0801101

Engels, H., and J. Wirth. 1997. "No Ergogenic Effects of Ginseng (Panax Ginseng C.A. Meyer) During Graded Maximal Aerobic Exercise." *Journal of the American Dietetic Association* 97, no. 10, pp. 1110–15. doi:10.1016/s0002-8223(97)00271-x

Engels, H., J. Said, and J. Wirth. 1996. "Failure of Chronic Ginseng Supplementation to Affect Work Performance and Energy Metabolism in Healthy Adults Female." *Nutrition Research* 16, no. 8, pp. 1295–305. doi:10.1016/0271-5317(96)00138-8

Felter, H.W., and J.U. Lloyd. 1898. *King's American Dispensatory.* Cincinnati, OH: The Ohio Valley Co.

Fendrick, A.M. 2003. "Viral Respiratory Infections Due to Rhinoviruses: Current Knowledge, New Developments." *American Journal of Therapeutics* 10, no. 3, pp. 193–202. doi:10.1097/00045391-200305000-00006

Forester, S., and J. Lambert. 2011. "Antioxidant Effects of Green Tea." *Molecular Nutrition & Food Research* 55, no. 6, pp. 844–54.

Foster, S. 1991. *Echinacea: Nature's Immune Enhancer.* Rochester, VT: Healing Arts Press.

Gebhardt, R. 1993. "Multiple Inhibitory Effects of Garlic Extracts on Cholesterol Biosynthesis in Hepatocytes." *Lipids* 28, no. 7, pp. 613–19. doi:10.1007/bf02536055

Gebhardt, R. 1995. "Amplification of Palmitate-Induced Inhibition of Cholesterol Biosynthesis in Cultured rat Hepatocytes by Garlic-Derived Organosulfur Compounds." *Phytomedicine* 2, no. 1, pp. 29–34. doi:10.1016/s0944-7113(11)80045-0

Gebhardt, R., H. Beck, and K. Wagner. 1994. "Inhibition of Cholesterol Biosynthesis by Allicin and Ajoene in Rat Hepatocytes and HepG2 cells." *Biochimica et Biophysica Acta* 1213, no. 1, pp. 57–62. doi:10.1016/0005-2760(94)90222-4

Geng, Z., and B.H.S. Lau. 1997. "Aged Garlic Extract Modulates Glutathione Redox Cycle and Superoxide Dismutase Activity in Vascular Endothelial Cells." *Phytotherapy Research* 11, no. 1, pp. 54–56. doi:10.1002/(sici)1099-1573(199702)11:1<54::aid-ptr950>3.3.co;2-p

Geng, Z., Y. Rong, and B.H.S. Lau. 1997. "S-Allyl Cysteine Inhibits Activation of Nuclear Factor Kappa B in Human T Cells." *Free Radical Biology Medicine* 23, no. 2, pp. 345–50. doi:10.1016/s0891-5849(97)00006-3

Gilmore, M.R. 1911. Bureau of American Ethnological Association's Annual Report.

Giunta, B., H. Hou, Y. Zhu, J. Salemi, A. Ruscin, R.D. Shytle, and J. Tan. 2010. "Fish Oil Enhances Anti-Amyloidogenic Properties of Green Tea EGCG in Tg2576 Mice." *Neuroscience Lettes* 471, no. 3, pp. 134–38. doi:10.1016/j.neulet.2010.01.026

Gonzalez-Seijo, J.C., Y.M. Ramos, and I. Lastra. 1995. "Manic Episode and Ginseng: Report of a Possible Case." *Journal of Clinical Psychopharmacology* 15, no. 6, pp. 447–48. doi:10.1097/00004714-199512000-00014

Gorski, J.C., S.M. Huang, A. Pinto, M.A. Hamman, J.K. Hilligoss, N.A. Zaheer, M. Desai, M. Miller, and S.D. Hall. 2004. "The Effect of Echinacea (Echinacea Purpurea Root) on Cytochrome P450 Activity in Vivo." *Clinical Pharmacology & Therapeutics* 75, no. 1, pp. 89–100. doi:10.1016/j.clpt.2003.09.013

Grimm, W., and H.H. Muller. 1999. "A Randomized Controlled Trial of the Effect of Fluid Extract of Echinacea Purpurea on the Incidence and Severity of Colds and Respiratory Infections." *The American Journal of Medicine* 106, no. 2, pp. 138–43. doi:10.1016/s0002-9343(98)00406-9

Grunwald, J., J. Heede, H.P. Koch, R. Albrecht, O. Knudsen, and N. Ramussen. 1992. "Effects of Garlic Powder Tablets on Blood Lipids and Blood Pressure—The Danish Multicenter Kwai(R) Study." *European Journal of Clinical Research* 3, pp. 179–86.

Gupta, N., and T.D. Porter. 2001. "Garlic and Garlic-Derived Compounds Inhibit Human Squalene Monooxygenase." *The Journal of Nutrition* 131, no. 6, pp. 1662–67.

Gurley, B.J., S.F. Gardner, and M.A. Hubbard. 2000. "Clinical Assessment of Potential Cytochrome P450-Mediated Herb-Drug Interactions." In AAPS Annual Meeting & Exposition, Indianapolis, IN.

Han, N., B. Liu, and M. Wang. 1992. "Effect of Allicin on Antioxidases in Mice." *Acta Nutrimenta Sinica* 14, pp. 107–8.

Harauma, A., and T. Moriguchi. 2006. "Aged Garlic Extract Improves Blood Pressure in Spontaneously Hypertensive Rats More Safely than Raw Garlic." *The Journal of Nutrition* 136, no. 3, pp. 769S–3S.

Hisano, M., H. Bruschini, A.C. Nicodemo, and M. Srougi. 2012. "Cranberries and Lower Urinary Tract Infection Prevention." *Clinics* 67, no. 6, pp. 661–67. doi:10.6061/clinics/2012(06)18

Holzgartner, H., U. Schmidt, and U. Kuhn. 1992. "Comparison of the Efficacy and Tolerance of a Garlic Preparation vs. Bezafibrate." *Arzneimittelforschung* 42, no. 12, pp. 1473–77.

Hong, B., Y.H. Ji, J.H. Hong, K.Y. Nam, and T.Y. Ahn. 2002. "A Double-Blind Crossover Study Evaluating the Efficacy of Korean Red Ginseng in Patients with Erectile Dysfunction: A Preliminary Report." *The Journal of Urology* 168, no. 5, pp. 2070–73. doi:10.1097/01.ju.0000034387.21441.87

Hudson, J.B. 2012. "Applications of the Phytomedicine Echinacea Purpurea (Purple Coneflower) in Infectious Diseases." *Journal of Biomedicine and Biotechnology* 2012: 769896. doi:10.1155/2012/769896

Ide, N., and B.H. Lau. 1999. "S-Allylcysteine Attenuates Oxidative Stress in Endothelial Cells." *Drug Development and Industrial Pharmacy* 25, no. 5, pp. 619–24. doi:10.1081/DDC-100102217

Ikeda, Y., A. Murakami, and H. Ohigashi. 2008. "Ursolic Acid: An Anti- and Pro-Inflammatory Triterpenoid." *Molecular Nutrition & Food Research* 52, no. 1, pp. 26–42. doi:10.1002/mnfr.200700389

Inoue-Choi, M., J.M. Yuan, C.S. Yang, D.J. Van Den Berg, M.J. Lee, Y.T. Gao, and M.C. Yu. 2010. "Genetic Association Between the COMT Genotype and Urinary Levels of Tea Polyphenols and Their Metabolites among Daily Green Tea Drinkers." *International Journal of Molecular Epidemiology and Genetics* 1, no. 2, pp. 114–23.

Jain, A.K., R. Vargas, S. Gotzkowsky, and F.G. McMahon. 1993. "Can Garlic Reduce Levels of Serum Lipids? A Controlled Clinical Study." *The American Journal of Medicine* 94, no. 6, pp. 632–35. doi:10.1016/0002-9343(93)90216-c

Jandke, J., and G. Spiteller. 1987. "Unusual Conjugates in Biological Profiles Originating from Consumption of Onions and Garlic." *Journal of Chromatography* 421, pp. 1–8. doi:10.1016/0378-4347(87)80373-0

Jang, D.J., M.S. Lee, B.C. Shin, Y.C. Lee, and E. Ernst. 2008. "Red Ginseng for Treating Erectile Dysfunction: A Systematic Review." *British Journal of Clinical Pharmacology* 66, no. 4, pp. 444–50. doi:10.1111/j.1365-2125.2008.03236.x

Jatoi, A., N. Ellison, P.A. Burch, J.A. Sloan, S.R. Dakhil, P. Novotny, W. Tan, T.R. Fitch, K.M. Rowland, C.Y. Young, and P.J. Flynn. 2003. "A Phase II Trial of Green Tea in the Treatment of Patients with Androgen Independent Metastatic Prostate Carcinoma." *Cancer* 97, no. 6, pp. 1442–46. doi:10.1002/cncr.11200

Jepson, R.G., and J.C. Craig. 2008. "Cranberries for Preventing Urinary Tract Infections." *Cochrane Database of Systematic Reviews* 23, no. 1: CD001321. doi:10.1002/14651858.CD001321.pub4

Jin, J.-S., M. Touyama, T. Hisada, and Y. Benno. 2012. "Effects of Green Tea Consumption on Human Fecal Microbiota with Special Reference to Bifidobacterium Species." *Microbiology and Immunology* 56, no. 11, pp. 729–39. doi:10.1111/j.1348-0421.2012.00502.x

Jones, B.D., and A.M. Runikis. 1987. "Interaction of Ginseng with Phenelzine." *Journal of Clinical Psychopharmacology* 7, no. 3, pp. 201–2. doi:10.1097/00004714-198706000-00030

Jurgens, T.M., A.M. Whelan, L. Killian, S. Doucette, S. Kirk, and E. Foy. 2012. "Green Tea for Weight Loss and Weight Maintenance in Overweight or Obese Adults." *Cochrane Database of Systematic Reviews* 12: CD008650. doi:10.1002/14651858.CD008650.pub2

Kandil, O., T. Abdullah, A.M. Tabuni, and A. Elkadi. 1988. "Potential Role of Allium Sativum in Natural Cytotoxicity." *Archives of AIDS Research* 1, pp. 230–31.

Kang, S., and H. Min. 2012. "Ginseng, the 'Immunity Boost': The Effects of Panax Ginseng on Immune System." *Journal of Ginseng Research* 36, no. 4, pp. 354–68. doi:10.5142/jgr.2012.36.4.354

Karsch-Volk, M., B. Barrett, D. Kiefer, R. Bauer, K. Ardjomand-Woelkart, and K. Linde. 2014. "Echinacea for Preventing and Treating the Common Cold." *Cochrane Database of Systematic Reviews* 2: CD000530. doi:10.1002/14651858.CD000530.pub3

Kennedy, D.O., C.F. Haskell, K.A. Wesnes, and A.B. Scholey. 2004. "Improved Cognitive Performance in Human Volunteers Following Administration of Guarana (Paullinia Cupana) Extract: Comparison and Interaction with Panax ginseng." *Pharmacology Biochemistry Behavior* 79, no. 3, pp. 401–11. doi:10.1016/j.pbb.2004.07.014

Khoo, C., M. Hullar, F. Li, K. Stepaniants, L. Levy, R. Roderick, and J. Lampe. 2010. "Effect of Cranberry Juice Intake on Human Gut Microbial Community and Urinary Metabolites in a Randomized, Placebo-Controlled Intervention." *The FASEB Journal* 24, no. 1(Meeting Abstract Supplement): 720.3.

Kiefer, D., and T. Pantuso. 2003. "Panax Ginseng." *American Family Physician* 68, no. 8, pp. 1539–42.

Kim, B.H., Y.G. Lee, T.Y. Park, H.B. Kim, M.H. Rhee, and J.Y. Cho. 2009. "Gensenoside Rp1, a Ginsenoside Derivative, Blocks Lipopolysaccharide-Induced Interleukin-1Beta Production via Suppression of the NF-kappaB Pathway." *Planta Medica* 75, no. 4, pp. 321–26. doi:10.1055/s-0028-1112218

Kim, D.H., J.H. Chung, J.S. Yoon, Y.M. Ha, S. Bae, E.K. Lee, K.J. Jung, M.S. Kim, Y.J. Kim, M.K. Kim, and H.Y. Chung. 2013. "Ginsenoside Rd Inhibits the Expressions of iNOS and COX-2 by Suppressing NF-kB in LPS-Stimulated RAW264.7 Cells and Mouse Liver." *Journal of Ginseng Research* 37, no. 1, pp. 54–63. doi:10.5142/jgr.2013.37.54

Koch, H.P., W. Jagerr, J. Hysek, and B. Korpert. 1992. "Garlic and Onion Extracts: in Vitro Inhibition of Adenosine Deaminase." *Phytotherapy Research* 6, no. 1, pp. 50–52. doi:10.1002/ptr.2650060113

Koscielny, J., D. Klussendorf, R. Latza, R. Schmitt, H. Radtke, G. Siegel, and H. Kiesewetter. 1999. "The Antiatherosclerotic Effect of Allium Sativum." *Atherosclerosis* 144 no. 1, pp. 237–49. doi:10.1016/S0021-9150(99)00060-X

Lambert, J.D., and C.S. Yang. 2003. "Mechanisms of Cancer Prevention by Tea Constituents." *The Journal of Nutrition* 133, no. 10, pp. 3262S–7S.

Lau, B.H.S., F. Lam, and R. Wang-Cheng. 1987. "Effect of an Odor-Modified Garlic Preparation on Blood Lipids." *Nutrition Research* 7, no. 2, pp. 139–49. doi:10.1016/S0271-5317(87)80026-X

Lau, B.H.S., T. Yamasaki, and D.S. Grindley. 1991. "Garlic Compounds Modulate Macrophage and T-Lymphocyte Functions." *Mol Biother* 3, no. 2, pp. 103–7.

Lawson, L.D. 1998. "Garlic: A Review of Its Medicinal Effects and Indicated Active Compounds." In *Phytomedicines of Europe: Chemistry and Biological Activity*, eds L. Lawson and R. Bauer, 176–209. Washington, DC: American Chemical Society.

Le Gal, M., P. Cathebras, and K. Struby. 1996. "Pharmaton(R) Capsules in the Treatment of Functional Fatigue: A Double-Blind Versus Placebo Evaluated by a New Methodology." *Phytotherapy Research* 10, no. 1, pp. 49–53. doi:10.1002/(sici)1099-1573(199602)10:1<49::aid-ptr772>3.0.co;2-m

Lee, Y.J., Y.R. Jin, W.C. Lim, W.K. Park, J.Y. Cho, S. Jang, and S.K. Lee. 2003. "Ginsenoside-Rb1 Acts as a Weak Phytoestrogen in MCF-7 Human Breast Cancer Cells." *Archives of Pharmacal Research* 26, no. 1, pp. 58–63. doi:10.1007/bf03179933

Lee, F.C., J.H. Ko, J.K. Park, and J.S. Lee. 1987. "Effects of Panax Ginseng on Blood Alcohol Clearance in Man." *Clinical and Experimental Pharmacology and Physiology* 14, no. 6, pp. 543–46. doi:10.1111/j.1440-1681.1987.tb01510.x

Lee, B.M., S.K. Lee, and H.S. Kim. 1998. "Inhibition of Oxidative DNA Damage, 8-OHdG, and Carbonyl Contents in Smokers Treated with Antioxidants (Vitamin E, Vitamin C, Beta-Carotene and Red Ginseng)." *Cancer Letters* 132, no. 1–2, pp. 219–27. doi:10.1016/s0304-3835(98)00227-4

Lee, J., E. Lee, D. Kim, J. Lee, J. Yoo, and B. Koh. 2009. "Studies on Absorption, Distribution and Metabolism of Ginseng in Humans After Oral Administration." *Journal of Ethnopharmacology* 122, no. 1, pp. 143–48. doi:10.1016/j.jep.2008.12.012

Li, J., and W. Zhong. 2014. "Ginsenoside Metabolite Compound K Promotes Recovery of Dextran Sulfate Sodium-Induced Colitis and Inhibits Inflammatory Responses by Suppressing NF-kappaB Activation." *PLoS One* 9, no. 2: e87810. doi:10.1371/journal.pone.0087810

Lu, H., X. Meng, and C.S. Yang. 2003. "Enzymology of Methylation of Tea Catechins and Inhibition of Catechol-O-Methyltransferase by (-)-Epigallocatechin Gallate." *Drug Metabolism Disposition* 31, no. 5, pp. 572–79. doi:10.1124/dmd.31.5.572

Mader, F.H. 1990. "Treatment of Hyperlipidemia with Garlic-Powder Tablets. Evidence from the German Association of General Practitioners' Multicenter Placebo-Controlled Double-Blind Study." *Arzneimittelforschung* 40, no. 10, pp. 1111–16.

Marchesi, J.R., D.H. Adams, F. Fava, G.D. Hermes, G.M. Hirschfield, G. Hold, M.N. Quraishi, J. Kinross, H. Smidt, K.M. Tuohy, L.V. Thomas, E.G. Zoetendal, and A. Hart. 2015. "The Gut Microbiota and Host Health: A New Clinical Frontier." *Gut*, pp. 1–10. doi:10.1136/gutjnl-2015-309990

Mateo-Carrasco, H., M.C. Galvez-Contreras, F.D. Fernandez-Gines, and T.V. Nguyen. 2012. "Elevated Liver Enzymes Resulting from an Interaction Between Raltegravir and Panax Ginseng: A Case Report and Brief Review." *Drug Metabolism and Drug Interactions* 27, no. 3, pp. 171–75. doi:10.1515/dmdi-2012-0019

Matsuura, H. 2001. "Saponins in Garlic as Modifiers of the Risk of Cardiovascular Disease." *The Journal of Nutrition* 131, no. 3, pp. 1000S–5S.

McElhaney, J.E., V. Goel, B. Toane, J. Hooten, and J.J. Shan. 2006. "Efficacy of COLD-fX in the Prevention of Respiratory Symptoms in Community-Dwelling Adults: A Randomized, Double-Blinded, Placebo Controlled Trial." *The Journal of Alternative Complementary Medicine* 12, no. 2, pp. 153–57. doi:10.1089/acm.2006.12.153

Miller, L.G. 1998. "Herbal Medicinals: Selected Clinical Considerations Focusing on Known or Potential Drug-Herb Interactions." *Archives of Internal Medicine* 158, no. 20, pp. 2200–11.

Miller, R.J., K.G. Jackson, T. Dadd, A.E. Mayes, A.L. Brown, J.A. Lovegrove, and A.M. Minihane. 2012. "The Impact of the Catechol-O-Methyltransferase Genotype on Vascular Function and Blood Pressure After Acute Green Tea Ingestion." *Molecular Nutrition & Food Research* 56, no. 6, pp. 966–75. doi:10.1002/mnfr.201100726

Muller-Jakic, B., W. Breu, A. Probstle, K. Redl, H. Greger, and R. Bauer. 1994. "In Vitro Inhibition of Cyclooxygenase and 5-Lipoxygenase by Alkamides from Echinacea and Achillea Species." *Planta Medica* 60, no. 1, pp. 37–40. doi:10.1055/s-2006-959404

Nagae, S., M. Ushijima, S. Hatono, J. Imai, S. Kasuga, H. matsuura, Y. Itakura, and Y. Higashi. 1994. "Pharmacokinetics of the Garlic Compound S-Allylcysteine." *Planta Medica* 60, no. 3, pp. 214–17. doi:10.1055/s-2006-959461

Nantz, M.P., C.A. Rowe, C.E. Muller, R.A. Creasy, J.M. Stanilka, and S.S. Percival. 2012. "Supplementation with Aged Garlic Extract Improves both NK and Gammadelta-T cell Function and Reduces the Severity of Cold and Flu Symptoms: A Randomized, Double-Blind, Placebo-Controlled Nutrition Intervention." *Clinical Nutrition* 31, no. 3, pp. 337–44. doi:10.1016/j.clnu.2011.11.019

National, Cancer Institute. November 17, 2010. "Tea and Cancer Prevention: Strengths and Limits of the Evidence." National Cancer Institute. http://www.cancer.gov/about-cancer/causes-prevention/risk/diet/tea-fact-sheet (accessed August 2, 2015).

Nocerino, E., M. Amato, and A.A. Izzo. 2000. "The Aphrodisiac and Adaptogenic Properties of Ginseng." *Fitoterapia* 71, no. Suppl 1, pp. S1–S5. doi:10.1016/S0367-326X(00)00170-2

Novotny, J.A., D.J. Baer, C. Khoo, S.K. Gebauer, and C.S. Charron. 2015. "Cranberry Juice Consumption Lowers Markers of Cardiometabolic Risk, Including Blood Pressure and Circulating C-Reactive Protein, Triglyceride, and Glucose Concentrations in Adults." *Journal of Nutrition* 145, no. 6, pp. 1185–93. doi:10.3945/jn.114.203190

Oh, K.J., M.J. Chae, H.S. Lee, H.D. Hong, and K. Park. 2010. "Effects of Korean Red Ginseng on Sexual Arousal in Menopausal Women: Placebo-Controlled, Double-Blind Crossover Clinical Study." *The Journal of Sexual Medicine* 7, no. 4Pt1, pp. 1469–77. doi:10.1111/j.1743-6109.2009.01700.x

Ong, W.Y., T. Farooqui, H.L. Koh, A.A. Farooqui, and E.A. Ling. 2015. "Protective Effects of Ginseng on Neurological Disorders." *Frontiers Aging Neuroscience* 7, p. 129. doi:10.3389/fnagi.2015.00129

Park, H.J., J.H. Lee, Y.B. Song, and K.H. Park. 1996. "Effects of Dietary Supplementation of Lipophilic Fraction from Panax Ginseng on cGMP and cAMP in Rat Platelets and on Blood Coagulation." *Biological & Pharmaceutical Bulletin* 19, no. 11, 1434–39. doi:10.1248/bpb.19.1434

Piscitelli, S.C., A.H. Burstein, N. Welden, K.D. Gallicano, and J. Falloon. 2002. "The Effect of Garlic Supplements on the Pharmacokinetics of Saquinavir." *Clinical Infectious Diseases* 34, no. 2, pp. 234–38. doi:10.1086/324351

Predy, G.N., V. Goel, R. Lovlin, A. Donner, L. Stitt, and T.K. Basu. 2005. "Efficacy of an Extract of North American Ginseng Containing Poly-Furanosyl-Pyranosyl-Saccharides for Preventing Upper Respiratory Tract Infections: A Randomized Controlled Trial." *Canadian Medical Association Journal* 173, no. 9, pp. 1043–48. doi:10.1503/cmaj.1041470

Rahman, K., and D. Billington. 2000. "Dietary Supplementation with Aged Garlic Extract Inhibits ADP-Induced Platelet Aggregation in Humans." *The Journal of Nutrition* 130, no. 11, pp. 2662–65.

Rasheed, N., E. Tyagi, A. Ahmad, K.B. Siripurapu, S. Lahiri, R. Shukla, and G. Palit. 2008. "Involvement of Monoamines and Proinflammatory Cytokines in Mediating the Anti-Stress Effects of Panax Quinquefolium." *Journal of Ethnopharmacology* 117, no. 2, pp. 257–62. doi:10.1016/j.jep.2008.01.035

Reay, J.L., D.O. Kennedy, and A.B. Scholey. 2005. "Single Doses of Panax Ginseng (G115) Reduce Blood Glucose Levels and Improve Cognitive Performance During Sustained Mental Activity." *Journal of Psychopharmacology* 19, no. 4, pp. 357–65. doi:10.1177/0269881105053286

Reay, J.L., D.O. Kennedy, and A.B. Scholey. 2006. "Effects of Panax Ginseng, Consumed with and Without Glucose, on Blood Glucose Levels and Cognitive Performance During Sustained 'Mentally Demanding' Tasks." *Journal of Psychopharmacology* 20, no. 6, pp. 771–81. doi:10.1177/0269881106061516

Reay, J.L., A.B. Scholey, and D.O. Kennedy. 2010. "Panax Ginseng (G115) Improves Aspects of Working Memory Performance and Subjective Ratings of Calmness in Healthy Young Adults." *Human Psychopharmacology* 25, no. 6, pp. 462–71. doi:10.1002/hup.1138

Reuter, H., H.P. Koch, and L. Lawson. 1996. *Garlic: The Science and Therapeutic Application of Allium Sativum L. and Related Species*. Baltimore, MD: Williams and Wilkins.

Salvati, G., G. Genovesi, L. Marcellini, P. Paolini, I. De Nuccio, M. Pepe, and M. Re. 1996. "Effects of Panax Ginseng C.A. Meyer Saponins on Male Fertility." *Panminerva Medica* 38, no. 4, pp. 249–54.

Scaglione, F., G. Cattaneo, M. Alessandria, and R. Cogo. 1996. "Efficacy and Safety of the Standardised Ginseng Extract G115 for Potentiating Vaccination Against the Influenza Syndrome and Protection Against the Common Cold." *Drugs Experimental and Clinical Research* 22, no. 2, pp. 65–72.

Scaglione, F., F. Ferrara, S. Dugnani, M. Falchi, G. Santoro, and F. Fraschini. 1990. "Immunomodulatory Effects of Two Extracts of Panax Ginseng C.A. Meyer." *Drugs Experimental and Clinical Research* 16, no. 10, pp. 537–42.

Schappert, S.M., and E.A. Rechtsteiner. 2008. Ambulatory Medical Care Utilization Estimates for 2006. National Health Statistics Reports; no. 8, Hyattsville, MD: National Center for Health Statistics.

Sendl, A., G. Elbl, B. Steinke, K. Redl, W. Breu, and H. Wagner. 1992. "Comparative Pharmacological Investigations of Allium Ursinum and Allium Sativum." *Planta Medica* 58, no. 1, pp. 1–7. doi:10.1055/s-2006-961378

Shah, S.A., S. Sander, C.M. White, M. Rinaldi, and C.I. Coleman. 2007. "Evaluation of Echinacea for the Prevention and Treatment of the Common Cold: A Meta-Analysis." *Lancet Infect Dis* 7, no. 7, pp. 473–80. doi:10.1016/S1473-3099(07)70160-3

Sharma, M., S.A. Anderson, R. Schoop, and J.B. Hudson. 2009. "Induction of Multiple Pro-Inflammatory Cytokines by Respiratory Viruses and Reversal by Standardized Echinacea, a Potent Antiviral Herbal Extract." *Antiviral Research* 83, no. 2, pp. 165–70. doi:10.1016/j.antiviral.2009.04.009

Sharma, S.M., M. Anderson, S.R. Schoop, and J.B. Hudson. 2010. "Bactericidal and Anti-Inflammatory Properties of a Standardized Echinacea Extract (Echinaforce): Dual Actions Against Respiratory Bacteria." *Phytomedicine* 17, no. 8–9, pp. 563–68. doi:10.1016/j.phymed.2009.10.022

Shen, T., J. Lee, M.H. Park, Y.G. Lee, H.S. Rho, Y.S. Kwak, M.H. Rhee, Y.C. Park, and J.Y. Cho. 2011. "Ginsenoside Rp1, a Ginsenoside Derivative, Blocks Promoter Activation of iNOS and COX-2 Genes by Suppression of an IKKbeta-Mediated NF-kB Pathway in HEK293 Cells." *Journal of Ginseng Research* 35, no. 2, pp. 200–28. doi:10.5142/jgr.2011.35.2.200

Shin, H.R., J.Y. Kim, T.K. Yun, G. Morgan, and H. Vainio. 2000. "The Cancer-Preventive Potential of Panax Ginseng: A Review of Human and Experimental Evidence." *Cancer Causes & Control* 11, no. 6, pp. 565–76. doi:10.1023/A:1008980200583

Sivam, G.P. 2001. "Protection Against Helicobacter Pylori and Other Bacterial Infections by Garlic." *The Journal of Nutrition* 131, no. 3s, pp. 1106S–8S.

Sivam, G.P., J.W. Lampe, B. Ulness, S.R. Swanzy, and J.D. Potter. 1997. "Helicobacter Pylori—In Vitro Susceptibility to Garlic (Allium sativum) Extract." *Nutrition and Cancer* 27, no. 2, pp. 118–21. doi:10.1080/01635589709514512

Smith, M., K.M. Lin, and Y.P. Zheng. 2001. "PIII-89 an Open Trial of Nifedipine-Herb Interactions: Nifedipine with St. John's Wort, Ginseng or Ginkgo Biloba." *Clinical Pharmacology & Therapeutics* 69, no. 2, p. P86.

Sorensen, H., and J. Sonne. 1996. "A Double-Masked Study of the Effects of Ginseng on Cognitive Functions." *Current Therapeutic Research* 57, no. 12, pp. 959–68. doi:10.1016/s0011-393x(96)80114-7

Sotaniemi, E.A., E. Haapakoski, and A. Rautio. 1995. "Ginseng Therapy in Non-Insulin-Dependent Diabetic Patients." *Diabetes Care* 18, no. 10, pp. 1373–75. doi:10.2337/diacare.18.10.1373

Steele, V.E., G.J. Kelloff, D. Balentine, C.W. Boone, R. Mehta, D. Bagheri, C.C. Sigman, S. Zhu, and S. Sharma. 2000. "Comparative Chemopreventive Mechanisms of Green Tea, Black Tea and Selected Polyphenol Extracts Measured by in Vitro Bioassays." *Carcinogenesis* 21, no. 1, pp. 63–67. doi:10.1093/carcin/21.1.63

Steiner, M., A.H. Khan, D. Holbert, and R.I.-S. Lin. 1996. "A Double-Blind Crossover Study in Moderately Hypercholesterolemic Men that Compared the Effect of Aged Garlic Extract and Placebo Administration on Blood Lipids." *The American Journal of Clinical Nutrition* 64, no. 6, pp. 866–70.

Steiner, M., and R.I.S. Lin. 1994. "Cardiovascular and Lipid Changes in Response to Aged Garlic Extract Ingestion [Abstract]." *Journal of the American College of Nutrition* 13, no. 5, p. 524.

Steiner, M., and W. Li. 2001. "Aged Garlic Extract, a Modulator of Cardiovascular Risk Factors: a Dose-Finding Study on the Effects of Age on Platelet Functions." *The Journal of Nutrition* 131, no. 3s, pp. 980S–4S.

Stimpel, M., A. Proksch, H. Wagner, and M.L. Lohmann-Matthes. 1984. "Macrophage Activation and Induction of Macrophage Cytotoxicity by Purified Polysaccharide Fractions from the Plant Echinacea Purpurea." *Infection and Immunity* 46, no. 3, pp. 845–49.

Van Schepdael, P. 1993. "The Effects on Capacity of Ginseng G115(R) in Sports of Endurance." *Acta Therapeutica* 19, pp. 337–47.

Vorberg, G., and B. Schneider. 1990. "Therapy with Garlic: Results of a Placebo-Controlled, Double-Blind Study." *British Journal of Clinical Practice Supplement* 44, no. 69, pp. 7–11.

Warden, B.A., L.S. Smith, G.R. Beecher, D.A. Balentine, and B.A. Clevidence. 2001. "Catechins are Bioavailable in Men and Women Drinking Black Tea Throughout the Day." *The Journal of Nutrition* 131, no. 6, pp. 1731–37.

Wei, X.Y., J.Y. Yang, J.H. Wang, and C.F. Wu. 2007. "Anxiolytic Effect of Saponins from Panax Quinquefolium in Mice." *Journal of Ethnopharmacology* 111, no. 3, pp. 613–38. doi:10.1016/j.jep.2007.01.009

Woelkart, K., W. Xu, Y. Pei, A. Makriyannis, R.P. Picone, and R. Bauer. 2005. "The Endocannabinoid System as a Target for Alkamides from Echinacea Angustifolia Roots." *Planta Medica* 71, no. 8, pp. 701–5. doi:10.1055/s-2005-871290

World Health Organization. 1999. "Radix Ginseng." In *WHO Monographs on Selected Medicinal Plants*, 168–82. Geneva, Switzerland: World Health Organization.

Yale, S.H., and I. Glurich. 2005. "Analysis of the Inhibitory Potential of Ginkgo Biloba, Echinacea Purpurea, and Serenoa Repens on the Metabolic Activity of Cytochrome P450 3A4, 2D6, and 2C9." *The Journal of Alternative Complementary Medicine* 11, no. 3, pp. 433–39. doi:10.1089/acm.2005.11.433

Yeh, Y.Y., R.I.S. Lin, S.M. Yeh, and S. Evans. 1995. "Cholesterol Lowering Effects of Aged Garlic Extract Supplementation on Free-Living Hypercholesterolemic Men Consuming Habitual Diets." *Journal of the American College of Nutrition* 13, p. 545.

Yeh, Y.Y., and S.M. Yeh. 1994. "Garlic Reduces Plasma Lipids by Inhibiting Hepatic Cholesterol and Triacylglycerol Synthesis." *Lipids* 29, no. 3, pp. 189–93. doi:10.1007/bf02536728

Yin, S.Y., W.H. Wang, B.X. Wang, K. Aravindaram, P.I. Hwang, H.M. Wu, and N.S. Yang. 2010. "Stimulatory Effect of Echinacea Purpurea Extract on the Trafficking Activity of Mouse Dendritic Cells: Revealed by Genomic and Proteomic Analyses." *BMC Genomics* 11, no. 1, p. 612. doi:10.1186/1471-2164-11-612

Zhang, Y., L. Lin, G.Y. Liu, J.X. Liu, and T. Li. 2014. "Pharmacokinetics and Brain Distribution of Ginsenosides After Administration of Sailuotong." *Zhongguo Zhong Yao Za Zhi* 39, no. 2, pp. 316–21.

Zhu, Y., W. Ling, H. Guo, F. Song, Q. Ye, T. Zou, D. Li, Y. Zhang, G. Li, Y. Xiao, F. Liu, Z. Li, Z. Shi, and Y. Yang. 2013. "Anti-Inflammatory Effect of Purified Dietary Anthocyanin in Adults with Hypercholesterolemia: A Randomized Controlled Trial." *Nutrition Metabolism and Cardiovascular Diseases* 23, no. 9, pp. 843–49. doi:10.1016/j.numecd.2012.06.005

CHAPTER 5

Survey of the 20 Most Common Dietary Supplements—Sports Nutrition and Weight Management

Overview

This chapter discusses the five most popular dietary supplements used for sports and weight management. These include protein powders for building muscle; energy drinks and hydration drinks for running faster, longer, and recovering faster after sport; and garcinia cambogia (GC) and green coffee bean extract for weight loss. We will discuss the sources, traditional uses, manufacturing, and consumption of the products. We will review the research that might be used to determine their efficacy as well as their safety.

Introduction

The list of ingredients that fall under sports supplements and weight management are all products that attract people who would not normally take a dietary supplement. That is because these products are taken by people who are not necessarily looking to "do something good for their health." The products sold as sports nutrition and weight management (i.e., weight loss) supplements are used by people who want their bodies to perform at a level above what is average or normal. Sports nutrition products are designed to help you respond to exercise in a way that helps you grow larger and stronger muscles or run faster or longer. Weight loss products are pretty straightforward. People use them because they think they will cause fat loss. All of these expectations are driven largely by the marketing claims for these products. In this chapter, we will discuss the top five products used as sports nutrition and weight loss.

Protein

Background

Protein is a macronutrient essential to all living organisms. Proteins are composed of chains of smaller units called amino acids. Amino acids are classified as essential, nonessential, and conditionally essential (Table 5.1). Essential amino acids cannot be produced by the body; therefore, these must come from the diet. Nonessential amino acids when absent from the diet can be produced by the body using other nitrogen sources. Conditionally, essential amino acids are normally not essential accept in times of metabolic, physiologic, or immunological stress.

Protein is used by the body as structural components of body tissues as well as enzymes, carriers, and antibodies. Protein in the diet comes primarily from animal sources and secondarily from vegetable sources save in the case of vegetarians. Protein rich foods include meat, poultry, fish, dairy, eggs, and to a lesser extent beans, legumes, grains, nuts and seeds. Dietary protein can also come from protein supplements. These are

Table 5.1 Classification of amino acids

Essential	Conditionally essential	Nonessential
histidine	arginine	alanine
isoleucine	cysteine	asparagine
leucine	glutamine	aspartic acid
lysine	glycine	glutamic acid
methionine	ornithine	
phenylalanine	proline	
threonine	serine	
tryptophan	tyrosine	
valine		

generally powders consisting of protein isolated from foods such as, milk, egg, soy, rice, and so on.

Dietary protein, whether it be foods or supplements, can be categorized not only by its source but also by its quality. Protein quality is a measure of a protein's ability to meet physiological needs. The less it takes to meet the body's needs, the higher the quality of the protein. Protein supplements can be further categorized as fast or slow, based on how long it takes to digest and absorb them.

Protein Quality

The simplest way to estimate the quality of a given protein is to break it down into its individual amino acids. Each protein food has different levels of essential and nonessential amino acids. The amino acid profile is then compared to a standard profile with an emphasis on essential amino acids. This is called "Chemical Scoring." Egg protein is the standard that is used in a chemical scoring scale for protein quality and has a rating of 100.

Although it is relatively easy and inexpensive to do a Chemical Scoring of any protein, it does not always accurately predict how well the body can utilize it.

Another way of expressing the quality of a protein is Biological Value (BV). BV scoring utilizes in vivo testing. In testing for BV, we measure how much nitrogen from a given protein is retained in the body after it is eaten. The final BV number derived using this formula:

$$BV = (\text{Nitrogen retained/Nitrogen absorbed}) \times 100.$$

The obvious advantage of this method over chemical scoring is that it can be done in vivo. There are a few problems with this method, however. First, there are interindividual physiological differences that can affect the results. Second, the test subject does not always represent the people that will be consuming the protein in the real world. Finally, just because nitrogen is being retained does not mean that it is being effectively utilized. There is considerable exchange of proteins among tissues that is hidden from view when only nitrogen intake and output are measured. One tissue could be lacking and a test of BV would not detect this.

Net Protein Utilization (NPU) is another test of protein quality. Like BV testing, NPU tests involve two nitrogen balance studies performed in animals. One involves measurements on zero protein intakes and the other on submaximal intake. The formula is:

$$NPU = (Nitrogen\ retained/Nitrogen\ intake) \times 100.$$

Its drawbacks are that if a low NPU is obtained, it is impossible to know if it is because of a poor amino acid profile or low digestibility.

One last test for protein quality is the Protein Efficiency Ratio (PER). PER is the best-known procedure for evaluating protein quality and is used in the United States as the basis for regulations regarding food labeling and for determining the Recommended Daily Intake (RDI) of a given protein. This method involves rats that are fed a measured amount of protein and weighed periodically as they grow. The PER is expressed as:

$$PER = weight\ gain\ (g)/protein\ intake\ (g).$$

The benefits of this method are its limited expense and simplicity. Its drawbacks are that it is time consuming; the amino acid needs of rats are not those of humans; and the amino acid needs of growing animals are not those of adult animals (e.g., growing animals and humans need more lysine).

As outlined previously, protein quality can be measured by the amino acid profile or ratio of the indispensable amino acids they contain. If a protein contains all the amino acids essential for life, it is called a "complete" protein and is given a high score on the Chemical Scoring test. Because some proteins are not as efficiently digested (bioavailable), there is a need to test for digestibility as well. This type of testing is called Protein Digestibility-Corrected Amino Acid Score (PDCAAS). The PDCAAS method is the standard used by the Food and Drug Administration (FDA) for classifying protein quality. The Food and Agricultural Organization (FAO) and the World Health Organization (WHO) also use the PDCAAS method for making protein intake recommendations. It is now a federally accepted standard for determining protein quality for preschool-aged children. PDCAA of a protein is calculated by the following equation:

PDCAAS = Lowest uncorrected amino acid score × protein digestibility.

Protein Supplements

Therefore, we now know how to classify proteins, but we still haven't covered the dizzying array of products currently on store shelves. Most of the available protein powders are high quality proteins. Because PDCAAS is the world standard for measuring protein quality, we will compare each of our protein supplement options using this scoring method.

The second important characteristic of protein is its absorption *rate*. Proteins are described as being either "fast" or "slow" based on how fast the amino acids from the meal enter the blood stream (Boirie et al. 1997; Dangin et al. 2001). Most all meats and solid dairy foods are slow proteins. Most (but not all) protein powders, because they are so easily digested, are fast proteins. This characteristic of protein will come into play as we discuss which protein to use in various situations. The first and most common protein powder supplement is milk protein.

Casein

Quality: PDCAAS = 1
Absorption: Slow
Nearly 80 percent of milk protein is in the form of casein. The rest, about 20 percent, is whey protein. The distinguishing property of casein is its low solubility in acidic environments, like your stomach. As a result, casein digests slowly and is absorbed at a relatively slow constant rate over a few hours after it is eaten. Casein comes in two varieties in most powdered formulation: as a caseinate or in its native micellar form. Caseinates are treated with acid, which makes them coagulate and bind with minerals such as calcium before they are dried. Micellar casein is obtained through a filtration process that leaves the protein in its original untreated form and not bound to minerals.

The structure of casein protein protects it against heat. This makes casein easy to use in baked goods. This same unique structure also makes casein insoluble in water. This has made it difficult to make pure casein supplements that mix instantly with water. If you remember the first milk protein powders years ago, they were virtually impossible to get to dissolve completely. Today they are used in combination with other proteins that dissolve more easily creating a "blend." Occasionally, manufacturers will "agglomerate" the casein. This creates an "instantized" powder that dissolves readily in water. Casein is nearly tasteless but is often described as having a bland or mild milky taste.

Whey

Quality: PDCAAS = 1

Absorption: Fast

Raw whey is the runny yellowish stuff that's left floating at the top of real yogurt as well as milk after it coagulates. Not too appetizing at this point. Whey that is used for dietary supplements is a byproduct of cheese manufacturing. Raw whey consists of about 94 percent water and 6 percent whey "solids." Of the raw whey solids, 75 percent is lactose, 14 percent is protein, and the remaining 11 percent is made up of minerals and fat. The primary proteins in whey are beta-lactoglobulins, alpha-lactalbumins, bovine serum albumin, and immunoglobulins. You may have seen these mentioned in the ingredients list on your tub of whey protein, though most manufacturers don't bother to list out the specific protein fractions.

Whey comes in three forms, concentrate, isolate, and hydrolysate. Whey protein concentrate is made by passing the liquid whey from cheese processing through pasteurization, a separator, and then ultrafiltration and diafiltration. Ultrafiltration and diafiltration is a process that uses semipermeable membranes to sequentially filter nonprotein components of raw whey until the desired concentration of protein is achieved. The resulting protein rich liquid is then dried through spray drying which removes most all of the water. Whey concentrate contains whey protein as well as some lactose, fat, and minerals. This is less expensive to produce than whey protein isolate because it requires fewer steps and common equipment during processing.

Whey protein isolate is just that, isolated whey proteins. Moisture, lactose, fat, and minerals are removed through an ion exchange processes leaving nearly 95 percent pure protein. This is higher than whey concentrate, which contains roughly 80 percent whey protein. You'll know you have some protein isolate if it foams up when using a blender or even some shaker bottles. Stir it briskly and let it sit for a moment and you'll see the foam rise to the top if it is really whey isolate. Whey protein concentrate may also make foam but only slightly. If you have a glass of what the manufactures claim is pure whey isolate and it doesn't foam, I would be suspicious. The reason I am going on about this is that some unscrupulous manufacturers have been known to use whey concentrate and advertise it as whey isolate and charge higher prices to increase their margins. Both whey concentrate and isolate have a bland if not slightly sweet taste.

Finally, some manufactures have put an additional twist on whey protein isolate, subjecting it to an enzymatic process that partially hydrolyzes or predigests the protein. This form of whey protein isolate is called whey protein hydrolysate. Whey hydrolysate has a very bitter taste and, for this reason, can only be used blended with other proteins and usually doesn't exceed more than 10 to 15 percent of the total. Again, if you find a product that is advertised as being any more than a small percentage whey hydrolysate and it still tastes good, I would be suspicious. Interestingly whey hydrolysate is commonly used in infant formulas, and it doesn't seem to bother them at all. Give whey hydrolysate to an adult, however, and they are likely to spit it out!

Egg White

Quality: PDCAAS = 1

Absorption: Fast

Powdered egg whites, though not as popular today as in years past, are also an excellent protein source. Egg white, sometimes called egg albumin, is used as the standard for protein quality when measured by chemical scoring. This is because of its favorable amino acid profile.

In the past, egg protein was difficult to use in powders because it does not mix easily with a spoon. It always left clumps. Today, like casein, egg protein can be instantized. You can also find egg protein powders that also contain some powdered yolk. Still, most protein powders containing egg are blended with casein and whey. Egg white protein has virtually no taste.

Soy Isolate

Quality: PDCAAS = 1
Absorption: Fast
Soy protein isolate is prepared by isolating the protein fraction of defatted soy flour. This creates a powder that is 90 to 95 percent pure protein. In the past, you could detect soy in a protein drink because it finished with a gritty mouth feel. Today, however, the texture of soy isolate has been refined and is barely noticeable. Soy is best known for its association with cholesterol metabolism. Many studies have demonstrated a beneficial effect of soy protein on cholesterol levels.

Soy protein isolate is often compared to whey protein isolate as a vegetarian alternative. Studies comparing the anabolic properties of whey and soy show whey is considerably more anabolic under "athletic training" conditions. This is explained in part by higher levels of the amino acid leucine found in whey protein isolate. Soy protein isolate has a mild "beany" taste.

Brown Rice Protein

Quality: PDCAAS = 1
Absorption: Fast
Brown Rice protein is a newcomer to the dietary supplement scene. People don't usually think of brown rice as a good source of protein. In fact, as a grain, brown rice is only 7 to 9 percent protein. That protein, however, when concentrated and isolated, yields a powder that is ~90 percent protein. Rice protein isolate is made from protein enriched rice flour. Through various enzymatic processes, an 85 to 91 percent protein powder is obtained. Brown rice protein has a mild almost sweet taste.

Hemp Protein Concentrate

Quality: PDCAAS =< 0.5
Absorption: Slow
Hemp protein, like rice protein, is relatively new to the protein powder list. Hemp protein is most commonly found as a concentrate. As

such it contains not only protein, but significant fiber and fat. Hemp protein isolate is prepared in a similar manner as soy isolate. Due to the excessive cost, hemp protein isolate is not as common and for the cost sensitive consumer, it may not be a "best buy." Hemp protein has a mild, yet hearty, nutty flavor.

Rationale for Supplementation

Achieving a Nutritionally Adequate Intake of Protein

Nutritional requirements in the United States are set by the Food and Nutrition Board, National Academy of Sciences and published as the Dietary Reference Intakes. The current Recommended Dietary Allowance (RDA) for protein is 0.8 g/kg (0.36 g/lb) of body weight per day. This assumes the source is a high quality protein comparable to milk protein. The recommendation is the same for adult men and nonpregnant women of all ages, including older adults. As an example, the RDA for a 150 pound individual is ~54 g protein per day. The current RDA for protein is believed to meet the needs of most (97 to 98 percent) of the healthy sedentary adult population.

Special Populations—Athletes and the Elderly.

The Estimated Average Requirement (EAR) and RDA are calculated based on the results of nitrogen-balance studies. Using this methodology, the EAR is determined to be the average *minimum* amount of protein (nitrogen) intake to balance nitrogen excretion and avoid progressive loss of body protein over time. The RDA, set at two standard deviations above the EAR (0.66 g/kg/day), is assumed to be sufficient to meet the dietary needs of nearly all healthy adults. However, rigorously controlled nitrogen-balance studies tend to be small. In addition, low-protein diets can induce metabolic adaptations that spare nitrogen, essentially masking protein insufficiency (Motil et al. 1981). The EAR then reflects not the required protein intake for optimal function but, instead, reflects a state of metabolic accommodation at the lowest tolerable protein intake to avoid deficiency. This has caused some to question the appropriateness of current protein intake recommendations (Elango et al. 2010; Volpi et al. 2013).

Athletes

Controversy has existed in academia concerning the need and safety of athletes consuming more than the RDA for protein. The RDA for protein in healthy adults, which has been previously discussed above is 0.8 g/kg body weight per day. The RDA for protein is likely not sufficient to compensate for the oxidation of protein or amino acids during exercise (approximately 1 to 5 percent of the total energy cost) nor is it sufficient to provide optimal support for muscle growth or for the repair of exercise-induced muscle damage. Research has shown that subjects go into a negative nitrogen balance for 14 to 21 days after beginning a new or unaccustomed strength training protocol. Protein intakes of 2.2 to 2.6 g/kg bodyweight are needed to keep strength training subjects in nitrogen balance when beginning a new or unaccustomed strength training protocol. This is three times the RDA for healthy adults.

The following seven points are quoted from the position stand of the International Society of Sports Nutrition on protein and exercise (Campbell et al. 2007):

1. Vast research supports the contention that individuals engaged in regular exercise training require more dietary protein than sedentary individuals.
2. Protein intakes of 1.4 to 2.0 g/kg/day for physically active individuals are not only safe, but may improve the training adaptations to exercise training.
3. When part of a balanced, nutrient-dense diet, protein intakes at this level are not detrimental to kidney function or bone metabolism in healthy, active persons.
4. While it is possible for physically active individuals to obtain their daily protein requirements through a varied, regular diet, supplemental protein in various forms are a practical way of ensuring adequate and quality protein intake for athletes.
5. Different types and quality of protein can affect amino acid bioavailability following protein supplementation. The superiority

of one protein type over another in terms of optimizing recovery and training adaptations remains to be convincingly demonstrated.

6. Appropriately timed protein intake is an important component of an overall exercise training program, essential for proper recovery, immune function, and the growth and maintenance of lean body mass.

7. Under certain circumstances, specific amino acid supplements, such as branched-chain amino acids (BCAA's), may improve exercise performance and recovery from exercise.

It must be acknowledged that not all modes of exercise impact protein energy requirements equally. Campbell et al. in their position stand on protein intake and exercise recommend that exercising individuals ingest protein ranging from 1.4 to 2.0 g/kg/day. Individuals engaging in endurance exercise should ingest levels at the lower end of this range, individuals engaging in intermittent activities should ingest levels in the middle of this range, and those engaging in strength or power exercise should ingest levels at the upper end of this range (Campbell et al. 2007).

Elderly

The concern about the adequacy of established protein requirements is magnified in populations such as the elderly (Campbell et al. 2001; Volpi et al. 2013). Data suggests that consistent ingestion of the RDA for protein results in *reduced* skeletal muscle size in weight-stable older adults, independent of muscle function. Add to this the prevalence of sarcopenia in older populations. Sarcopenia is a syndrome characterized by progressive and generalized loss of skeletal muscle mass and strength. Sarcopenia represents an impaired state of health with a high personal toll—mobility disorders, increased risk of falls and fractures, impaired ability to perform activities of daily living, disabilities, loss of independence, and increased risk of death.

In cases of sarcopenia, the RDA for protein may not be enough to counter the pathology of sarcopenia. Data from the Health, Aging and Body Composition cohort study indicate that a lower protein intake in healthy older adults is associated with a larger loss of lean body mass over a period of 3 years. More recent data from the InCHIANTI study and the Women's Health Initiative cohort studies report the same findings, supporting the suggestion that a higher protein intake than the established recommendations is associated with reduced loss of muscle mass and reduced risk of strength loss and incident frailty (Beasley et al. 2010).

Weight Management

High protein diets can improve both appetite and ability to prevent weight regain following weight loss. Protein-rich meals (~25 to 30 g protein) are known to increase thermogenesis (i.e., body heat production) and reduce appetite. Higher-protein diets lead to greater body weight loss, fat loss, and protect muscle mass compared to lower protein diets. Improvements in select cardiometabolic health markers are also often improved. High protein diets can work long term as long as compliance to the diet is maintained. For a high protein diet to work, at least 1.2 and 1.6 g protein/kg/day should be included with at least 25 to 30 g of protein per meal (Leidy et al. 2015). Protein supplements can be used to achieve this level of dietary protein and should be consumed with a solid meal whenever possible. Also, "slow" proteins such as casein may provide better results than fast proteins such as whey or soy protein.

Safety

There is a common misconception that "Too much protein stresses the kidney." A secondary claim that protein increases calcium excretion and increases the risk of osteoporosis is also often used as an argument against higher protein intake. Both claims are unfounded as there is no substantive evidence that high protein intakes at the levels discussed in this chapter will have any adverse effects on healthy individuals (Martin, Armstrong, and Rodriguez 2005). Individuals with pre-existing mild renal insufficiency need to closely monitor their kidney status with the guidance of their physician or health care provider as observational data from epidemiological studies provide evidence both for and against dietary protein restriction in cases of kidney disease (Johnson 2006; Martin, Armstrong, and Rodriguez 2005).

Energy Drinks

Background

Caffeine is possibly the most popular drug in the world. The United States is the world's largest consumer of energy drinks by volume, reaching roughly 290 million gallons in 2007 (Higgins, Tuttle, and Higgins 2010). In 2010, energy drink sales totaled $20 per capita, equal to approximately one-half the sales of sugar-sweetened sodas and surpassing sales of both sports drinks and fruit drinks (Harris and Munsell 2015). In 2012, sales of energy drinks reached $6.9 billion, and sales of newly introduced "energy shots" totaled $1.1 billion, reflecting increases of 19 and 9 percent, respectively, over the previous year. In the midst of declining sale for most sugary drinks, including soda, from 2007 to 2012, gallon sales of energy drinks increased by 53 percent (Harris and Munsell 2015). When energy drink marketers extol the desirable attributes of their products to Americans, they are singing to the choir.

Energy drinks are sold as both beverages and dietary supplements. Caffeine is considered both a food additive and a drug according to the Federal Drug Administration (U.S. FDA 2007). The difference under DSHEA is subtle, having to do with whether or not a product claims to be a "dietary supplement" and if the product has a supplement facts panel or a nutrition facts panel. How the product is packaged, what is on the label, the serving size and ingredients, all contribute to the determination of whether or not a product is a beverage or a dietary supplement (FDA 2015).

Energy drinks are similar to soft drinks in that they are carbonated and come with or without sugar. Energy drinks differ from caffeinated soft drinks in the amount of caffeine that they contain. Whereas soft drinks and "colas" contain from 22 mg of caffeine on the low end to 55 mg on the high end, energy drinks start at 80 mg and go as high as 210 mg caffeine per serving (Sorkin et al. 2014). Energy drinks also differ in that they tend to contain more active ingredients. These are usually the amino acid taurine, B vitamins, and various herbal extracts such as guarana, ginseng, and ginkgo biloba. These added ingredients allow the various products to differentiate themselves, but research fails to support the claim that they do anything that high doses of caffeine is not already doing for (or to) the consumer.

Caffeine is a methyxanthine. As such, it possesses a number of properties that most people are familiar with. Caffeine is a stimulant and acts as a sympathomimetic. Although caffeine has shown the ability in vitro to inhibit phosphodiesterase and interact with the sympathetic nervous system, the majority of caffeine's effects can be attributed to its ability to block adenosine receptors (Ribeiro and Sebastião 2010). Adenosine's role in the body, generally speaking, is to suppress arousal and induce sleep. Caffeine, acting as an adenosine receptor blocker, produces the opposite effects. Even though the primary action of caffeine may be to block adenosine receptors, because of the multiple roles of adenosine in the brain, this leads to very important secondary effects on many different neurotransmitters, including noradrenaline, dopamine, serotonin, acetylcholine, glutamate, and gamma aminobutyric acid (GABA) (Fredholm et al. 1999). This in turn influences a large number of different physiological functions.

Taurine is a popular active ingredient used by energy drink marketers. One popular energy drink's name is a play on the word taurine. Taurine got its name from the source from which it was first isolated, ox bile, Taurus being Latin for "bull." Taurine, a sulfur-containing beta-amino acid (2-aminoethanesulphonic acid) is regarded as a conditionally essential amino acid. Taurine is produced in the liver and the brain and plays an important role as an antioxidant in osmolarity regulation, muscle contraction, and neuroprotection. The question is does taurine add any energy benefits to energy drinks? It has been suggested that taurine may enhance physical performance because of its role in skeletal muscle. In vitro studies and studies in animals have shown that artificially increasing muscle taurine levels above normal can enhance the twitch characteristics of fast twitch muscle. Human studies however have shown that supplementing with taurine for 7 days does not affect taurine levels within skeletal muscle (Galloway et al. 2008). Taurine appears to be tightly regulated in both skeletal muscle and brain, making the idea of altering intracellular levels of taurine through supplementation unlikely.

B vitamins are water-soluble vitamins required as coenzymes for proper cell function. They are included in energy drinks because of their role in metabolism and the production of energy from carbohydrates. B vitamins include thiamine (B1), riboflavin (B2), niacin (B3), pantothenic acid (B5), pyridoxine hydrochloride (B6), biotin (B7), inositol (formerly B8), and cyanocobalamin (B12). A brief description of each should suffice.

Thiamine (vitamin B1) is essential for the proper function of the citric acid cycle and serves as a coenzyme in carbohydrate metabolism.

Riboflavin (vitamin B2) plays an important role in the respiratory chain of mitochondria and is involved in energy metabolism involving fats, carbohydrates, and proteins.

Niacin (vitamin B3) is required for the production of nicotinamide adenine dinucleotide (NADH), which is required for energy production through oxidative phosphorylation. NADH also supports the production of neurotransmitters such as dopamine, serotonin, and norepinephrine.

Pantothenic acid (vitamin B5) is required for production of Krebs cycle intermediates as well as fatty acid oxidation.

Pyridoxine hydrochloride (vitamin B6) is a coenzyme involved in amino acid and homocysteine metabolism, glucose and lipid metabolism, neurotransmitter production, and DNA and RNA synthesis.

Biotin (vitamin B7) is the coenzyme required for gluconeogenesis and fatty acid oxidation. Inositol exists in nine possible stereoisomers but the most common form in the body is myo-inositol. It is part of cell membranes, plays a role in helping the liver process fats, and contributes to the function of muscles and nerves.

Vitamin B12 is involved in the cellular metabolism of carbohydrates, proteins, and lipids. It also helps maintain nerve cell function, is needed for production of DNA, and is important for production of red blood cells.

Although B vitamins are involved enzymatically in energy metabolism in the body, they are not stimulants or sympathomimetic. Their inclusion in energy drinks is more marketing than physiology. Claims that "B vitamins give you energy" are misleading in that the claims are made in the context of "feeling" increased energy after consuming them. This does not occur, and if most people would reflect on their experience taking a multivitamin for example, they would realize that taking a multivitamin (which includes B vitamins) does not give you the sensation of increased energy. Likewise, taking B vitamins do not produce the sensation of energy.

Guarana (*Paullinia cupana*) is a vine that grows native in the Amazon rain forest of South America. The vine has been domesticated by Amazonians who prize its fruit for its rich caffeine content. Guarana contains about four times as much caffeine as coffee. In fact, guarana seeds contain more caffeine than any other plant in the world, with levels ranging from 2 to ~8 percent; guarana also contains other stimulants in the xanthine group like theobromine and theophylline (Smith and Atroch 2010). Guarana can add a meaningful amount of caffeine if included in the formula for an energy drink. Often time, however, the guarana and other herbal extracts are listed as part of a proprietary "energy blend" (Higgins, Tuttle, and Higgins 2010). If being marketed as a dietary supplement, proprietary blends may be used to disclose the individual ingredients without having to disclose the exact amounts. For this reason, the actual amount of caffeine in a product could exceed the amount added as pure caffeine.

Ginseng is a popular herb used not only in energy drinks but also as standalone herbal extract products. Ginseng has been traditionally used for thousands of years as an adaptogen, meaning it is thought to help the body cope with stress. The active component of ginseng are called ginsenosides. Standardized ginseng ginsenoside content ranges from 1 to 7 percent. Energy drinks however, do not normally list the ginsenoside content, and it would be expected that they also do not use the more expensive standardized extract form of the herb. Like guarana, ginseng is usually included as part of a proprietary "energy blend" without disclosing the actual amount the product contains per serving. It is uncertain if most products contain an efficacious amount of ginseng to provide any adaptogenic benefits.

G. biloba is another herb with a long history of traditional use for cognitive performance. In vitro and animal studies have confirmed ginkgo's properties as an antioxidant. It may also offer some protection to nerve cells from oxidative stress. There is also some evidence that it may possess properties that might support cardiovascular health through its antioxidant, antiplatelet, antithrombotic, vasodilatory, and antihypertensive properties (Rabito and Kaye 2013). Research falls equally for and against support for claims of ginkgo providing cognitive benefit to healthy individuals. To date, no large, well-conducted randomized controlled trials have shown that it has predictable and meaningful benefits in healthy persons beyond serving as an antioxidant.

Finally, what about caffeine and taurine together? Perhaps it is the combination that provides some benefits over caffeine alone? A crossover study (i.e., each subject experienced each of the different treatment conditions at different times separated by a "washout" period) conducted in 2010 looked at the effect of caffeine and taurine alone and in combination on the locomotor activity of rats (Dombovy-Johnson 2012). No significant differences were seen between caffeine and caffeine plus taurine on rat locomotor behavior. The authors concluded the data provides results that "justify the inclusion of caffeine in energy drinks, but does not provide evidence for a synergistic relationship between caffeine and taurine" (Dombovy-Johnson 2012). In a previous placebo-controlled study of the effects of a popular energy drink containing both caffeine and taurine on high-intensity run time-to-exhaustion in physically active university students did not influence high-intensity run time-to-exhaustion (Candow et al. 2009). This is in agreement with a more recent study in soldiers consuming caffeine, taurine, or the combination before tests of physical and cognitive performance (Kammerer 2014). In should be noted that the placebo did not contain caffeine or taurine. However, in a study of twelve trained cyclists, improved cycling time-trial performance was noted after ingestion of a caffeine and taurine containing energy drink (Ivy et al. 2009). Once again, the placebo used in this study did not contain caffeine or taurine. After all is said and done, there is little evidence that the combination of caffeine with taurine offers anything that caffeine alone does not provide as far as "energy" is concerned.

Safety

In 2011, the American Academy of Pediatrics issued a report that raised significant concerns about the consumption of energy drinks by youth; quoting from the report, "rigorous review and analysis of the literature reveal that caffeine and other stimulant substances contained in energy drinks have no place in the diet of children and adolescents

(American Academy of Pediatrics 2011; Harris and Munsell 2015)."
The concern is not just for youth. A number of concerning adverse
event reports following energy drink consumption have been published
(Higgins, Tuttle, and Higgins 2010). Four documented cases of caffeine-
associated death have been reported, as well as five separate cases of sei-
zures associated with consumption of energy drinks (Clauson et al. 2003).
A healthy 28-year-old man had cardiac arrest after a day of drinking large
amounts of energy drinks and motocross racing. A healthy 18-year-old
man died playing basketball after drinking two cans of Red Bull. Postural
tachycardia associated with a vasovagal reaction was reported in a young
volleyball player after an excess intake of a popular energy drink, leading
experts to suspect the drink as a possible cause of orthostatic intolerance.
Finally, four cases of psychiatric effects on patients with known psychiatric illness were reported. It is not unreasonable to assume that these
adverse effects are attributable to excess caffeine intake.

Although the FDA has not made official comment on the safety of
energy drinks, a review authored by Dr. John P. Higgins and colleagues
published in the journal *Mayo Clinic Proceedings* offers some sensible
precautions (Higgins, Tuttle, and Higgins 2010):

- Limit intake of energy drinks to no more than one can per day.
- Use water to rehydrate during and after exercise.
- Do not consume energy drinks if you have high blood
  pressure.
- Report any adverse events you may experience as a result of
  taking an energy drink.
- Do not mix energy drinks with alcohol.
- If you have any pre-existing medical condition, consult your
  physician or health care provider before using energy drinks.
- For athletes participating in events lasting less than one hour,
  they recommend against the use of energy drinks because of
  possible negative cardiovascular effects. Use water instead.
- For athletes participating in events lasting more than one
  hour, they recommend against the use of energy drinks.
  Choose instead electrolyte based beverages formulated
  specifically for restoring fluid balance.

Garcinia Cambogia

Background

GC is the scientific name for Malabar tamarind, a plant with small bitter fruit native to Southeast Asia. The small fruits are about 5 cm in diameter with 6 to 8 grooves like tiny gourds. The rind of the fruit is traditionally used in Asian countries as a food preservative and flavoring agent. The dried and smoked rind of the fruit is an important spice in India and parts of Asia with its cultivation and trade being economically noteworthy. It is also used as a traditional medicine as treatment for joint pain, digestive problems, and other common ailments. The rind is also used in industrial settings as a substitute for acetic acid in latex manufacturing (Semwal et al. 2015).

Rationale for Supplementation

The primary reason GC is used as a dietary supplement is for weight loss. Hydroxycitric acid (HCA) is the major organic acid occurring in the GC fruit, and the major active ingredient used in dietary supplements. In vitro, HCA inhibits adenosine triphosphate (ATP)-citrate lyase, the enzyme responsible for catalyzing the extra mitochondrial cleavage of citrate to oxaloacetate and acetyl-coenzyme A (acetyl-CoA), a building block of fatty acid synthesis (Watson and Lowenstein 1970). In other words, HCA has the ability to block an enzyme that the body uses to convert sugar into fat (a.k.a. de novo lipogenesis) (Kovacs and Westerterp-Plantenga 2006). The logic then follows that if you block conversion of sugar into fat in your body, then you should gain less fat from excess carbohydrates in your diet. That is the logic anyway. The clinical trials assessing its ability to help people lose weight, however, have not been as straightforward.

Many of the weight loss studies involving GC have used a combination of herbal extracts and other ingredients. Because there is no way of knowing what impact GC had on the outcome of those studies, they will not be included in our discussion. Instead, we will focus on those studies using only GC extract. Let us begin chronologically. The earliest study that the author is aware of is a 1996 study done on 35 healthy subjects

(Roman, Flores, and Alarcon 1996). This 8 week study included calorie restricted diets plus 1,500 mg GC daily. Subjects taking GC reported reduced appetite and experienced a reduction in bodyweight. It should be noted that if the mechanism of action of GC is the inhibition of lipogenesis from excess carbohydrates by HCA, a calories restricted diet would, in and of itself, reduce de novo lipogenesis. So studies involving calorie restriction make the results difficult to interpret.

Two years following the study by Roman, Heymsfield et al. published the results of a double blind placebo controlled trial of GC in 84 overweight men and women (Heymsfield et al. 1998). Subjects were put on a high-fiber low calorie diet for 12 weeks. In addition, 42 subjects were given 1,500 mg HCA in the form of a GC extract and the remaining 42 subjects were given placebo. Subjects in both groups lost a significant amount of weight during the 12 weeks; however, there was no difference in weight loss between the GC group and the placebo. GC also had no effect on the composition of body weight lost during the 12 weeks. Again, using a low calorie or calorie-restricted diet creates a big uncontrolled variable that can invalidate claims that GC has an impact on weight loss.

Two studies were published in 2000. One acute study gave 18 g of HCA to endurance-trained subjects during a single bout of endurance exercise to see if there was any effects on substrate utilization (van Loon et al. 2000). No differences were seen between GC and placebo on fat oxidation, carbohydrate oxidation, or respiratory exchange ratio. Again, the mechanism of GC should theoretically reduce weight gain by a reduction in de novo lipogenesis. It is difficult to see how this mechanism would improve endurance performance, and unsurprisingly it did not in this study.

That same year Mattes et al. published a double blind placebo controlled study in which 89 mildly overweight females were put on a 1,200 kcal/day diet for 12 weeks to see if HCA had any impact on appetite (Mattes and Bormann 2000). Forty-two subjects were given 2,400 mg GC extract per day providing 1,200 mg HCA. Both groups lost weight with the GC group achieving a small yet significantly greater reduction. Those in the GC group reported no difference in appetite or ease at sticking with the diet than placebo.

A pair of studies were published in 2001, neither showing improved weight loss compared to placebo. Both were 2-week crossover studies, measuring weight loss and energy expenditure alone or in combination, with medium-chain triglycerides (MCT) (Kovacs et al. 2001; Kovacs, Westerterp-Plantenga, and Saris 2001). Neither weight loss or energy expenditure was effected by GC consumption (500 mg HCA) with or without MCTs. This same group published another crossover trial in 2002 demonstrating that 300 mg HCA taken for two weeks was able to reduce food intake in 24 overweight subjects eating in a laboratory setting (Westerterp-Plantenga and Kovacs 2002).

In 2003, Hayamizu et al. conducted a 12-week double-blind place-bo-controlled trial in 39 subjects with central obesity (i.e., excess abdom-inal fat storage) (Hayamizu et al. 2003). Subjects were given 1,000 mg HCA per day. Measures were taken after 8 weeks and again 4 weeks after HCA supplementation had been discontinued. Subjects receiving HCA experienced significantly reduced abdominal fat mass but did not differ from placebo in body-mass index (BMI) or amount of weight lost.

The last clinical trial we will look at is a 2011 double-blind placebo control trial of GC in overweight subjects. Eighty-six overweight subjects were to maintain their normal diet, and then they were randomly assigned to receive GC (2 g/day) or placebo for 10 weeks (Kim et al. 2011). *Garcinia* supplementation failed to promote weight loss or any clinically significant change in body composition (% body fat). Additionally, GC had no effect on triglycerides, cholesterol, fat cell signaling, or antioxidant status. A meta-analysis completed this same year determined that after controlling for methodological design, dose, and outliers, no significant difference could be seen in weight loss with GC (Onakpoya et al. 2011).

As can be seen by our review of available evidence of the effectiveness of GC for weight loss, there are a number of factors that make inter-preting the data difficult. For one, if the mechanism responsible for GC influencing bodyweight is by inhibiting de novo lipogenesis, then putting trail subjects on a calorie-restricted diet removes the impact of anything reducing the conversion of excess carbohydrates into fat. Many trials also involved instruction on various forms of physical activity. Granted, reducing calories and increasing physical activity is the right thing to do if you want to lose weight. Including this in studies trying to isolate the weight loss effects of an herbal supplement, however, is at least counter-productive. Add to that including studies that use a blend of different herbal extracts and an assortment of vitamins and minerals muddies the waters, so to speak. In the end, GC should theoretically be most effective as a measure to reduce body fat gain while on a high carbohydrate diet (Kovacs and Westerterp-Plantenga 2006).

Safety

Garcinia has been used traditionally for centuries without adversely affecting the health of those who consume it. Nevertheless, when used as a dietary supplement, levels of active compounds can be consumed in much higher levels compared to traditional use. For this reason, it is important to examine the potential adverse effects of its use as a dietary supplement. A published review of the safety of GC included 13 nonacute studies that analyzed the effects of supplementing with HCA isolated from GC (Márquez et al. 2012). In total 930 subjects were included in the analysis. On average, the amount of GC extract used in the studies ranged between 1,500 and 4,667 mg/day providing between 900 and 2,800 mg/day of HCA. Liver and reproductive effects and general adverse health effects were included. Collectively, no differences were found in humans in terms of side effects or adverse events between groups taking GC extracts and the placebo groups at the doses used. Additionally, the raw material has been submitted for generally recognized as safe (GRAS) status to the FDA without objection.

Green Coffee

Background

The green coffee extract dietary supplement is made from the raw, unroasted seeds of the *Coffea* fruits, also referred to as coffee berries or coffee cherries. Coffee is best grown in areas of the world around the equatorial zone, commonly referred to as "The Bean Belt." The species of *Coffea* used for this supplement include *C. Arabica*, *C. canephora*

(*C. robusta, C. bukobensis*), and *C. liberica* (*C. arnoldiana*). The chemical composition of green coffee is complex, providing hundreds of different compounds, each of which has the potential to provide independent effects in the body. The most well-known compound is caffeine, a stimulant from the methylxanthine family. Other methylxanthines found in Green Coffee beans include theobromine and theophylline (Franzke et al. 1968). Chlorogenic acids, catechol-containing plant polyphenols, are also part of the green coffee bean make up. Green coffee also contains the polysaccharides arabinogalactans, glactomannans and cellulose, epicatechin, catechin, ferulic acid, cafeoyltryptophan, rutin, the triterpene esters kehweol and cafestol, and the amino acids alanine and asparagine.

Chlorogenic acids are the compounds in green coffee believed most responsible for the health benefits associated with the ingredient. Coffee beans have among the highest levels of chlorogenic acids compared with other plants, and chlorogenic acids accumulate in the beans as they ripen. The roasting process used in the production of coffee beans for the popular beverage reduces the amount of chlorogenic acid in the bean (Farah et al. 2005). Therefore, green coffee has higher chlorogenic acid levels that roasted coffee beans. The main chlorogenic acids in green coffee include the hydroxycinnamic acid derivatives caffeoylquinic acids, dicaffeoylquinic acids, and feruloylquinic acids (Iwai et al. 2004).

As a dietary supplement, green coffee bean is sometimes offered as a standardized extract, standardized to a percentage of chlorogenic acid. This percentage usually ranges from approximately 30 to 50 percent. These ingredients are also sometimes standardized to a specific caffeine content as well. Some green coffee extracts are decaffeinated, while others do not remove the caffeine. Chlorogenic acids from green coffee extracts are easily absorbed. It appears chlorogenic acid is absorbed across the digestive tract, with early absorption occurring in the stomach and jejunum followed by absorption along the small intestine and even later in the large intestine (Farah et al. 2008).

In the body, chlorogenic acid has effects on enzymes that can affect blood glucose levels. Studies show chlorogenic acid inhibits the glucose-6-phosphate transporter T1, a transporter protein on glucose-6-phosphatase, resulting in reduced hepatic glucose output (Arion et al.

1997; Herling et al. 1999). Further studies report, chlorogenic acids in decaffeinated coffee were believed to decrease glucose-dependent insulinotropic polypeptide and increase glucagon-like peptide 1 secretion resulting in decreased glucose transport and decreased intestinal glucose absorption rates (Johnston, Clifford, and Morgan 2003).

Components of green coffee also have reported anti-inflammatory activity in the body. The diterpenes kahweol and cafestol suppress the LPS-induced production of prostaglandin E(2), COX-2 protein and mRNA expression, and COX-2 promoter activity in a dose-dependent manner. Prostaglandin E2 plays a key role in the resolution of inflammation. Kahweol has also blocked the LPS-induced activation of NF-kappaB by preventing IkappaB degradation and inhibiting IkappaB kinase activity (Kim, Jung, and Jeong 2004). NF-kappa B is an inflammatory protein chronically active in many inflammatory diseases.

Coffee, and to a greater extent green coffee also have well-established antioxidant and antifree radical activity (Daglia et al. 2000; Ramalakshmi, Kubra, and Rao 2007). The chlorogenic acid found in green coffee extracts is shown to have the highest antioxidant activity is 5-caffeoylquinic acid (Fujioka and Shibamoto 2006). Green coffee and chlorogenic acid alone have both been shown to reduce hydrogen peroxide-induced DNA damage (Glei et al. 2006). Kahweol and cafestol, other compounds in green coffee have been reported to support the activity of glutathione, the major endogenous antioxidant enzyme in the body (Lam, Sparnins, and Wattenberg 1982).

Rationale for Supplementation

The most common motivation for supplementation with green coffee extract is to promote weight loss. Greater than two-thirds of adults and one-third of children and adolescents in the United States are overweight or obese (Flegal et al. 2012; Ogden et al. 2012). A large percentage of these individuals are trying to lose weight, and many of them are turning to dietary supplements to help them in the process. This has created an immensely successful sector of the dietary supplement market valued at $2 billion per year. A few clinical trials have studied the effects of green coffee bean supplementation on weight loss. In a meta-analysis, three studies observing the effect of green coffee extract on weight loss were reviewed. These studies provided green coffee extract ranging in dosages from 180 to 200 mg/day for 4 to 12 weeks. The results showed a statistically significant reduction in body weight with green coffee extract as compared with placebo, indicating the supplement is able to support weight loss in overweight individuals (Onakpoya, Terry, and Ernst 2011). However, the authors of the meta-analysis reported several limitations of the studies reviewed including small sample sizes, unclear dosages used, short duration, and unclear blinding policies, reducing the overall strength of the studies reviewed.

Green coffee extract is also used to support healthy blood pressure levels. The antihypertensive benefits of this supplement are believed due to a possible effect of ferulic acid on muscarinic acetylcholine receptors (Suzuki et al. 2002). A clinical trial of several doses of a standardized green coffee extract ranging from 46 to 185 mg/day evaluated the dose response effect of the supplement in healthy individuals with mildly elevated blood pressure. Results of the study found a dose-dependent significant improvement in blood pressure levels versus placebo (Kozuma et al. 2005). As with most dietary supplements, long-term intake of the green coffee extract was necessary for the benefit to occur.

Safety

Green coffee extract is safe when taken orally and at the appropriate recommended dosages. Although some green coffee extracts are decaffeinated, there are some that do contain caffeine. Therefore, for those individuals who have a caffeine sensitivity, attention should be paid to the caffeine dosage provided in different green coffee extracts so as not to exceed dosages that do not exacerbate their condition.

There are Moderate Interaction Ratings for the combination of green coffee extract with alcohol, alendronate (Fosamax), anticoagulant, and antiplatelet drugs including aspirin, clopidogrel (Plavix), dipyridamole (Persantine), ticlopidine (Ticlid), ardeparin (Normiflo), dalteparin (Fragmin), enoxaparin (Lovenox), heparin and warfarin, beta-adrenergic agonists including albuterol (Ventolin, Proventil), metaproterenol (Alupent), terbutaline (Brethine, Bricanyl) and isoproterenol (Isuprel), closapine (Closaril), disulfiram (Antabuse), ephedrine, estrogens, fluvoxamine (Luvox), monoamine oxidase inhibitors (MAOIs), pentobarbital (Nembutal), phenylpropanolamine, quinolone antibiotics (Cipro, Penetrex, Tequin, Levaquin, Maxaquin, Avelox, Noroxin, Floxin, Zagam, and Trovan), riluzole (Rilutek), stimulants, theophylline, and verapamil (Calan, Covera, Isoptin, Verelan) (Natural Medicines 2015). Consumers should be cautious with these combinations.

Hydration Drinks

Background

Water makes up a large percentage of the human body, approximately 73 percent of lean body mass, and is essential for optimal physiological function and health (Sawka and Coyle 1999). This body water is the necessary medium for biochemical reactions, provides transportation of solutes throughout the body, supplies nutrients, and removes waste. Under normal circumstances, humans drink enough water to maintain adequate body water balance. However, there are times when the ability to maintain water balance may become more difficult, for example, heat or extreme cold exposure, altitude, increased respiration and urination, diarrheal diseases, and participation in sport or exercise, may make it difficult to balance fluid replacement with fluid losses, resulting in dehydration. It has been shown that all physiological systems in the body are detrimentally affected by dehydration (Murray 1995). During exercise, the body works to balance heat production and heat accumulation with heat dissipation using conduction, convection, evaporation, and radiation (Werner 1993). Evaporation is the principle process the body uses to promote heat loss during exercise, especially in hot, dry conditions, where it can account for as much as 98 percent of the body's cooling process (Armstrong and Maresh 1993). If rehydration is not sufficient to offset water loss through evaporation, progressive dehydration will result. Inadequate hydration can lead to detrimental effects on health and performance. Dehydration of only 1 to 2 percent of body weight can result in compromised physiological function and athletic performance. If dehydration is allowed to continue to losses greater than 3 percent of body weight, it can result in an increased risk for exertional heat illnesses including heat cramps, heat exhaustion, or even heat stroke.

Water loss due to sweating is accompanied by a loss of electrolytes, predominantly sodium. The amount of sodium lost during exercise depends upon sweating rate and duration and the concentration of sodium in the individual's sweat. Sweat sodium concentrations can range from 15 to 90 mmol/L, with an average of approximately 40 mmol/L (Baker et al. 2009). Even those athletes with low sweat sodium concentrations can lose a substantial amount of sodium with long periods of strenuous exercise or high sweating rates. Sweat sodium concentration can also be affected by hydration status. Although sodium is the chief electrolyte in sweat, chloride, potassium, calcium, and magnesium are also lost in perspiration.

There are numerous detrimental effects of dehydration on the body. Dehydration leads to an increase in core temperature during exercise. With every one percent of body weight lost to sweat, there is a subsequent 0.15°C to 0.20°C increase in core temperature (Sawka et al. 1985). In addition, dehydration can lead to increased cardiovascular strain indicated by decreased stroke volume, increased heart rate, increased systemic vascular resistance, lower cardiac output, and mean arterial pressure, and these changes are proportional to water losses (Gonzalez-Alonso et al. 1995). Dehydration also leads to changes in muscle tissue, including a decreased rate of glycogen degradation, elevated muscle temperature, and increased lactate levels (Casa, Maresh, and Armstrong 2000; Edwards et al. 1972; Hargeaves et al. 1996). Dehydration can also affect the mental function of athletes, resulting in increased perceived exertion ratings and decreased motivation and time to exhaustion (Gopinthan, Pichan, and Sharma 1988). Effects of dehydration on athletic performance are also documented in the research. Performance decrements include reductions in high-intensity endurance, run-time to exhaustion, maximal aerobic power, oxygen consumption, and execution of sport-specific skills (Burge, Carey, and Payne 1993; Caldwell, Ahonen, and Nousiainen 1984; Dougherty et al. 2006; Judelson et al. 2007; Pinchan et al. 1988).

The simplest rehydration strategy is drinking water, but optimal rehydration beverages often also include carbohydrates and electrolytes to improve taste, stimulate thirst, accelerate intestinal fluid absorption, and promote fluid retention by the body. These other ingredients may also help promote physical performance during the rehydration process. Several physical characteristics of hydration beverages can influence the acceptance of the beverage, and in turn, its proper use, including salinity, color, sweetness, temperature, flavor, carbonation, and viscosity (Passe, Horn, and Murray 1997; Wilk and Bar-Or 1996; Wilk et al. 1998). Including carbohydrates and electrolytes in these beverages may also help maintain blood glucose levels, carbohydrate oxidation, and electrolyte balance, which are also important for athletic performance.

Timing of consumption may also affect the ability of a hydration beverage to support optimal performance. Thirst is not a good indicator of hydration status, as the sensation is delayed compared with the physiological indicators of dehydration. Therefore, it is important that athletes drink fluids before feeling thirsty to maintain optimal hydration status. It is recommended that athletes consume 500 mL of fluid 2 hours before exercising (Convertino et al. 1996). Hydration in the 24 hours prior to exercise is also important for overall performance. Some research supports overhydrating prior to exercise in the heat to enhance thermoregulatory function and limit potential performance decrements due to dehydration. Proper hydration during exercise is also very important. Hydrating during exercise bouts helps to conserve the centrally circulating fluid volume to allow for adequate heat dissipation, cardiac output, perfusion of working muscles, and evaporative cooling.

While consuming fluids is necessary for hydration, gastric emptying, intestinal absorption, and retention of the fluids and electrolytes are also critical for optimal hydration. Absorption of water is minimal in the stomach, therefore fluids must get past the stomach and into the small intestine for absorption to occur. Higher rates of gastric emptying are encouraged with high gastric volume through water or dilute carbohydrate solutions. In the intestines, fluid uptake is inversely impacted by beverage composition including carbohydrate content and osmolality. Once absorbed into the bloodstream, the fluid needs to be retained and, therefore, needs to be formulated to avoid diuresis.

Ingredients other than water can be included in hydration beverages to support absorption and retention, as well as provide ergogenic aids for improved physical performance. Common ingredients include carbohydrate, electrolytes, protein, and stimulants. Carbohydrates serve the dual purpose in hydration beverages of absorption and blood glucose level support. The cotransport of glucose and sodium facilitate the passive absorption of water in the intestines. Electrolytes added to hydration beverages can also improve palatability and stimulate the drive to drink. Athletes may not feel thirsty in the early stages of dehydration, so stimulating the drive to drink may help increase overall fluid consumption. Once absorbed, increased sodium concentrations and osmolality can stimulate renal water reabsorption, and the osmolyte properties of sodium can help maintain extracellular fluid volume. Protein may be included in hydration beverages as an ergogenic aid to promote muscle protein synthesis. It may also support plasma volume expansion and thermoregulatory adaptation through promoting albumin synthesis (Goto et al. 2010). Stimulants, such as caffeine, are also added to hydration beverages occasionally for their ergogenic benefits. Stimulants can prevent central fatigue, improve mood, support cognitive function, and improve physical performance.

Rationale for Supplementation

The principal rationale for consuming hydration drinks is to avoid the detrimental effects of dehydration and electrolyte loss on athletic performance, to supplement energy levels during exercise, and to replace fluid lost during exercise. According to The American College of Sports Medicine and the Institute of Medicine, hydration drinks consumed during exercise should contain 20 to 30 mmol/L of sodium and 2 to 5 mmol/L of potassium (Institute of Medicine 1994; Sawka et al. 2007). These concentrations of sodium in hydration drinks is shown to stimulate physiological thirst and improve palatability and voluntary fluid intake, and the combination of sodium and potassium helps replace sweat losses from exercise (Wilk and Bar-Or 1996). Sodium losses are also associated with muscle cramping, which may be avoided by consuming these sodium levels in hydration drinks (Bergeron 2003). Furthermore, the presence of sodium in hydration drinks helps stimulate more complete rehydration by supporting better plasma volume restoration and whole-body fluid balance following exercise. Expert panels recommend that athletes should drink 1.5 L of a sodium-containing fluid for each kg of body mass lost to achieve rapid and complete recovery from dehydration. Carbohydrates are added to these beverages as a source of energy, but also to slow gastric emptying. It is reported that a relatively dilute carbohydrate solution, up to 6 percent or 60 g/L allow for stomach emptying at a similar rate equal to water (Murray 1987). Higher concentrations of carbohydrate can impair gastric emptying leading to an increase in gastrointestinal discomfort. The type of carbohydrate used may also influence the overall benefit provided by a hydration drink. A 2:1 ratio of glucose and fructose has been shown to increase gastric emptying and fluid absorption versus glucose alone (Jeukendrup and Moseley 2010). These effects are important to the athlete because the glucose from carbohydrate is the primary substrate for contracting muscles during exercise, and maintaining carbohydrate levels during exercise is an effective strategy for delaying fatigue and improving endurance capacity (Coyle et al. 1983). Inclusion of carbohydrate in hydration drinks is also shown to impact fluid retention following exercise-induced dehydration (Evans, Shirreffs, and Maughan 2009).

Safety

Hydration drinks are generally safe. Beverages with higher carbohydrate levels than those outlined in the preceding may result in gastrointestinal upset due to delayed gastric emptying, but these effects are transient. For those individuals with a sensitivity to caffeine, caution should be used when consuming hydration beverages with added caffeine.

References

American Academy of Pediatrics. 2011. "Sports Drinks and Energy Drinks for Children and Adolescents: Are They Appropriate?" *Pediatrics* 127, no. 6, pp. 1182–89. doi:10.1542/peds.2011-0965

Arion, W.J., W.K. Canfield, F.C. Ramos, P.W. Schindler, H.J. Burger, H. Hemmerle, G. Schubert, P. Below, and A.W. Herling. 1997. "Chlorogenic Acid and Hydroxynitrobenzaldehyde: New Inhibitors of Hepatic Glucose 6-Phosphatase." *Archives of Biochemistry and Biophysics* 339, no. 2, pp. 315–22. doi:10.1006/abbi.1996.9874

Armstrong, L.E., and C.M. Maresh. 1993. "The Exertional Heat Illnesses: A Risk of Athletic Participation." *Medicine Exercise Nutrition Health* 2, pp. 125–134.

Baker, L.B., J.R. Stofan, A.A. Hamilton, and C.A. Horswill. 2009. "Comparison of Regional Patch Collection vs. Whole Body Washdown for Measuring Sweat Sodium and Potassium Loss During Exercise." *Journal of Applied Physiology* 107, no. 3, pp. 887–95. doi:10.1152/japplphysiol.00197.2009

Beasley, J.M., A.Z. LaCroix, M.L. Neuhouser, Y. Huang, L. Tinker, N. Woods, Y. Michael, J.D. Curb, and R.L. Prentice. 2010. "Protein Intake and Incident Frailty in the Women's Health Initiative Observational Study." *Journal of American Geriatrics Society* 58, no. 6, pp. 1063–71. doi:10.1111/j.1532-5415.2010.02866.x

Bergeron, M.F. 2003. "Heat Cramps: Fluid and Electrolyte Challenges During Tennis in the Heat." *Journal Science and Medicine in Sport* 6, no. 1, pp. 19–27. doi:10.1016/s1440-2440(03)80005-1

Boirie, Y., M. Dangin, P. Gachon, M.P. Vasson, J.L. Maubois, and B. Beaufrère. 1997. "Slow and Fast Dietary Proteins Differently Modulate Postprandial Protein Accretion." *Proceedings of National Academy of Sciences* 94, no. 26, pp. 14930–35. doi:10.1073/pnas.94.26.14930

Burge, C.M., M.F. Carey, and W.R. Payne. 1993. "Rowing Performance, Fluid Balance, and Metabolic Function Following Dehydration and Rehydration." *Medicine & Science Sports & Exercise* 25 no. 12, pp. 1358–64. doi:10.1249/00005768-199312000-00007

Caldwell, J.E., E. Ahonen, and U. Nousiainen. 1984. "Differential Effects of Sauna-, Diuretic-, and Exercise-Induced Hypohydration." *Journal of Applied Physiology Respiratory Environmental and Exercise Physioogyl* 57, no. 4, pp. 1018–23.

Campbell, B., R.B. Kreider, T. Ziegenfuss, P. La Bounty, M. Roberts, D. Burke, J. Landis, H. Lopez, and J. Antonio. 2007. "International Society of Sports Nutrition Position Stand: Protein and Exercise." *Journal of Internatinal Society of Sports Nutrition* 4, no. 1, p. 8. doi:10.1186/1550-2783-4-8

Campbell, W.W., T.A. Trappe, R.R. Wolfe, and W.J. Evans. 2001. "The Recommended Dietary Allowance for Protein May Not Be Adequate for Older People to Maintain Skeletal Muscle." *The Journals of Gerontology Series A: Biological Sciences and Medical Sciences* 56, no. 6, pp. M373–78. doi:10.1093/gerona/56.6.m373

Candow, D.G., A.K. Kleisinger, S. Grenier, and K.D. Dorsch. 2009. "Effect of Sugar-Free Red Bull Energy Drink on High-Intensity Run Time-to-Exhaustion in Young Adults." *Journal of Strength and Conditioning Research* 23, no. 4, pp. 1271–75. doi:10.1519/jsc.0b013e3181a026c2

Casa, D.J., C.M. Maresh, and L.E. Armstrong. 2000. "Intravenous Versus Oral Rehydration During a Brief Period: Responses to Subsequent Exercise in the Heat." *Medicine and Science in Sports and Exercise* 32, no. 1, 124–33. doi:10.1097/00005768-200001000-00019

Clauson, K.A., K.M. Shields, C.E. McQueen, and N. Persad. 2003. "Safety Issues Associated with Commercially Available Energy Drinks." *Journal of American Pharmacists Association* 43, no. 3, pp. e55–63. doi: 10.1331/japha.2008.07055

Convertino, V.A., L.E. Armstrong, E.F. Coyle, G.W. Mack, M.N. Sawka, L.C. Senay Jr., and W.M. Sherman. 1996. "American College of Sports Medicine Position Stand. Exercise and Fluid Replacement." *Medicine and Science in Sports & Exercise* 28 no. 1, pp. i–vii. doi:10.1249/00005768-198410000-00017

Coyle, E.F., J.M. Hagberg, B.F. Hurley, W.H. Martin, A.A. Ehsani, and J.O. Holloszy. 1983. "Carbohydrate Feeding During Prolonged Strenuous Exercise can Delay Fatigue." *Journal of Applied Physiology* 55 no. 1, pp. 230–35.

Daglia, M., A. Papetti, C. Gregotti, F. Berte, and G. Gazzani. 2000. "In Vitro Antioxidant and Ex Vivo Protective Activities of Green and Roasted Coffee." *Journal of Agricultural and Food Chemistry* 48, no. 5, pp. 1449–54. doi:10.1021/jf990510g

Dangin, M., Y. Boirie, C. Garcia-Rodenas, P. Gachon, J. Fauquant, P. Callier, O. Ballèvre, and B. Beaufrère. 2001. "The Digestion Rate of Protein Is an Independent Regulating Factor of Postprandial Protein Retention." *American Journal of Physiology Endocrinology Metabolism* 280, no. 2, pp. E340–48.

Dombovy-Johnson, M. 2012. "The Effects of Taurine and Caffeine Alone and in Combination on Locomotor Activity in the Rat." *Colgate Academic Review* 7, no. 1, Article 10. http://commons.colgate.edu/car/vol7/iss1/10

Dougherty, K.A., L.B. Baker, M. Chow, and W.L. Kenney. 2006. "Two Percent Dehydration Impairs and Six Percent Carbohydrate Drink Improves Boys Basketball Skills." *Medicine & Science in Sports & Exercise* 38 no. 9, pp. 1650–58. doi:10.1249/01.mss.0000227640.60736.8e

Edwards, R.H.T., R.C. Harris, E. Hultman, L. Kaizer, D. Koh, and L. Nordesjo. 1972. "Effect of Temperature on Muscle Energy Metabolism and Endurance During Successive Isometric Contractions, Sustained to Fatigue, of the Quadriceps Muscle in Man." *The Journal of Physiology* 220, no. 2, pp. 335–52. doi:10.1113/jphysiol.1972.sp009710

Elango, R., M.A. Humayun, R.O. Ball, and P.B. Pencharz. 2010. "Evidence that Protein Requirements Have Been Significantly Underestimated." *Current Opinion in Clinical Nutrition and Metabolic Care* 13, no. 1, pp. 52–57. doi:10.1097/mco.0b013e328332f9b7

Evans, G.H., S.M. Shirreffs, and R.J. Maughan. 2009. "Postexercise Rehydration in Man: The Effects of Osmolality and Carbohydrate Content of Ingested Drinks." *Nutrition* 25, no. 9, pp. 905–13. doi:10.1016/j.nut.2008.12.014

Farah, A., M. Monteiro, C.M. Donangelo, and S. Lafay. 2008. "Chlorogenic Acids from Green Coffee Extract are Highly Bioavailable in Humans." *Journal of Nutrition* 138, no. 12, pp. 2309–15. doi:10.3945/jn.108.095554

Farah, A., T. de Paulis, L.C. Trugo, and P.R. Martin. 2005. "Effect of Roasting on the Formation of Chlorogenic Acid Lactones in Coffee." *Journal of Agricultural and Food Chemistry* 53, no. 5, pp. 1505–13. doi:10.1021/jf048701t

FDA. April 2015. "Guidance for Industry: Distinguishing Liquid Dietary Supplements from Beverages." *U.S. Food and Drug Administration: Protecting and Promoting your Health.* www.fda.gov/downloads/Food/GuidanceRegulation/GuidanceDocumentsRegulatoryInformation/DietarySupplements/UCM381220.pdf (accessed August 2015).

Flegal, K.M., M.D. Carroll, B.K. Kit, and C.L. Ogden. 2012. "Prevalence of Obesity and Trends in the Distribution of Body Mass Index Among US Adults, 1999–2010." *JAMA: The Journal of the American Medical Association* 307, no. 5, pp. 491–97. doi:10.1001/jama.2012.39

Franzke, C., K.S. Grunert, U. Hildebrandt, and H. Griehl. 1968. "On the Theobromine and Theophylline Content of Raw Coffee and Tea." *Pharmazie* 23, no. 9, pp. 502–3.

Fredholm, B.B., K. Bättig, J. Holmén, A. Nehlig, and E.E. Zvartau. 1999. "Actions of Caffeine in the Brain with Special Reference to Factors that Contribute to Its Widespread Use." *Pharmacological Reviews* 51, no. 1, pp. 83–133.

Fujioka, K., and T. Shibamoto. 2006. "Quantitation of Volatiles and Nonvolatile Acids in an Extract from Coffee Beverages: Correlation with Antioxidant Activity." *Journal of Agricultural and Food Chemistry* 54, no. 16, pp. 6054–58. doi:10.1021/jf060460x

Galloway, S.D., J.L. Talanian, A.K. Shoveller, G.J. Heigenhauser, and L.L. Spriet. 2008. "Seven Days of Oral Taurine Supplementation Does Not Increase Muscle Taurine Content or Alter Substrate Metabolism During Prolonged Exercise in Humans." *Journal of Applied Physiology* 105, no. 2, pp. 643–51. doi:10.1152/japplphysiol.90525.2008

Glei, M., A. Kirmse, N. Habermann, C. Persin, and B.L. Pool-Zobel. 2006. "Bread Enriched with Green Coffee Extract has Chemoprotective and Antigenotoxic Activities in Human Cells." *Nutrition and Cancer* 56, no. 2, pp. 182–92. doi:10.1207/s15327914nc5602_9

Gonzalez-Alonso, J., R. Mora-Rodriguez, P.R. Below, and E.F. Coyle. 1995. "Dehydration Reduces Cardiac Output and Increases Systemic and Cutaneous Vascular Resistance During Exercise." *Journal of Applied Physiology* 79, no. 5, pp. 1487–96.

Gopinthan, P.M., G. Pichan, and V.M. Sharma. 1988. "Role of Dehydration in Heat Stress-Induced Variations in Mental Performance." *Archives of Environmental Health* 43, no. 1, pp. 15–17. doi:10.1080/00039896.1988. 9934367

Goto, M., K. Okazaki, Y. Kamijo, S. Ikegawa, S. Masuki, K. Miyagawa, and H. Nose. 2010. "Protein and Carbohydrate Supplementation during 5-day Aerobic Training Enhanced Plasma Volume Expansion and Thermoregulatory Adaptation in Young Men." *Journal of Applied Physiology* 109, no. 4, pp. 1247–55. doi:10.1152/japplphysiol.00577.2010

Hargeaves, M., P. Dillo, D. Angus, and M. Febbraio. 1996. "Effect of Fluid Ingestion on Muscle Metabolism during Prolonged Exercise." *Journal of Applied Physiology* 80, no. 1, pp. 363–66.

Harris, J.L., and C.R. Munsell. 2015. "Energy Drinks and Adolescents: What's the Harm?" *Nutrition Reviews* 73, no. 4, pp. 247–57. doi:10.1093/nutrit/nuu061

Hayamizu, K., Y. Ishii, I. Kaneko, M. Shen, Y. Okuhara, N. Shigematsu, H. Tomi, M. Furuse, G. Yoshino, and H. Shimasaki. 2003. "Effects of Garcinia Cambogia (Hydroxycitric Acid) on Visceral Fat Accumulation: A Double-Blind, Randomized, Placebo-Controlled Trial." *Current Therapeutic Research Clinical Experimental* 64, no. 8, pp. 551–67. doi:10.1016/j.curtheres.2003.08.006

Herling, A.W., H. Burger, G. Schubert, H. Hemmerle, H. Schaefer, and W. Kramer. 1999. "Alterations of Carbohydrate and Lipid Intermediary Metabolism During Inhibition of Glucose-6-Phosphatase in Rats." *European Journal of Pharmacology* 386, no. 1, pp. 75–82. doi:10.1016/s0014-2999(99)00748-7

Heymsfield, S.B., D.B. Allison, J.R. Vasselli, A. Pietrobelli, D. Greenfield, and C. Nunez. 1998. "Garcinia Cambogia (Hydroxycitric Acid) as a Potential Antiobesity Agent: A Randomized Controlled Trial." *JAMA: The Journal of the American Medical Association* 280, no. 18, pp. 1596–600. doi:10.1001/jama.280.18.1596

Higgins, J.P., T.D. Tuttle, and C.L. Higgins. 2010. "Energy Beverages: Content and Safety." *Mayo Clinic Proceedings* 85, no. 11, pp. 1033–41.

Institute of Medicine. 1994. *Fluid Replacement and Heat Stress*. Washington, DC: National Academies Press.

Ivy, J.L., L. Kammer, Z. Ding, B. Wang, J.R. Bernard, Y.H. Liao, and J. Hwang. 2009. "Improved Cycling Time-Trial Performance After Ingestion of a Caffeine Energy Drink." *International Journal of Sport Nutrition and Exercise Metabolism* 19, no. 1, pp. 61–78.

Iwai, K., N. Kishimoto, Y. Kakino, K. Mochida, and T. Fujita. 2004. "In Vitro Antioxidative Effects and Tyrosine Inhibitory Activities of Seven Hydroxycinnamoyl Derivatives in Green Coffee Beans." *Journal of Agricultural and Food Chemistry* 52, no. 15, pp. 4893–98. doi:10.1021/jf040048m

Jeukendrup, A.E., and L. Moseley. 2010. "Multiple Transportable Carbohydrates Enhance Gastric Emptying and Fluid Delivery." *Scandinavian Journal of Medicine & Science in Sports* 20, no. 1, pp. 112–21. doi: 10.1111/j.1600-0838.2008.00862.x

Johnson, D.W. 2006. "Dietary Protein Restriction as a Treatment for Slowing Chronic Kidney Disease Progression: The Case Against." *Nephrology* 11, no. 1, pp. 58–62. doi:10.1111/j.1440-1797.2006.00550.x

Johnston, K.L., M.N. Clifford, and L.M. Morgan. 2003. "Coffee Acutely Modifies Gastrointestinal Hormone Secretion and Glucose Tolerance in Humans: Glycemic Effects of Chlorogenic Acid and Caffeine." *The American Journal of Clinical Nutrition* 78, no. 4, pp. 728–33.

Judelson, D.A., C.M. Maresh, J.M. Anderson, L.E. Armstrong, D.J. Casa, W.J. Kraemer, and J.S. Volek. 2007. "Hydration and Muscular Performance: Does Fluid Balance Affect Strength, Power and High-Intensity Endurance?" *Sports Medicine* 37, no. 10, pp. 907–21. doi:10.2165/00007256-200737100-00006

Kammerer, M., J.A. Jaramillo, A. García, J.C. Calderón, and L.H. Valbuena. 2014. "Effects of Energy Drink Major Bioactive Compounds on the Performance of Young Adults in Fitness and Cognitive Tests: A Randomized Controlled Trial." *Journal of the International Society of Sports Nutrition* 11, no. 1, pp. 44. doi:10.1186/s12970-014-0044-9

Kim, J.E., S.M. Jeon, K.H. Park, W.S. Lee, T.S. Jeong, R.A. McGregor, and M.S. Choi. 2011. "Does Glycine Max Leaves or Garcinia Cambogia Promote Weight-Loss or Lower Plasma Cholesterol in Overweight Individuals: A Randomized Control Trial." *Nutrition Journal* 10, no. 1, p. 94. doi:10.1186/1475-2891-10-94

Kim, J.Y., K.S. Jung, and H.G. Jeong. 2004. "Suppressive Effects of the Kahweol and Cafestol on Cyclooxygenase-2 Expression in Macrophages." *FEBS Letters* 569, no. 1–3, pp. 321–26. doi:10.1016/j.febslet.2004.05.070

Kovacs, E.M., and M.S. Westerterp-Plantenga. 2006. "Effects of (-)-Hydroxycitrate on Net Fat Synthesis as De Novo Lipogenesis." *Physiology Behavior* 88, no. 4–5, pp. 371–81. doi:10.1016/j.physbeh.2006.04.005

Kovacs, E.M., M.S. Westerterp-Plantenga, and W.H. Saris. 2001. "The Effects of 2-Week Ingestion of (--)-Hydroxycitrate and (--)-Hydroxycitrate Combined with Medium-Chain Triglycerides on Satiety, Fat Oxidation, Energy Expenditure and Body Weight." *International Journal of Obesity Related Metabolic Disorders* 25, no. 7, pp. 1087–94. doi:10.1038/sj.ijo.0801605

Kovacs, E.M., M.S. Westerterp-Plantenga, M. de Vries, F. Brouns, and W.H. Saris. 2001. "Effects of 2-Week Ingestion of (-)-Hydroxycitrate and (-)-Hydroxycitrate Combined with Medium-Chain Triglycerides on Satiety and Food Intake." *Physiology Behavior* 74, no. 4–5, pp. 543–49. doi:10.1016/s0031-9384(01)00594-7

Kozuma, K., S. Tsuchiya, J. Kohori, T. Hase, and I. Tokimitsu. 2005. "Antihypertensive Effect of Green Coffee Bean Extract on Mildly Hypertensive Subjects." *Hypertens Research* 28, no. 9, pp. 711–18. doi:10.1291/hypres.28.711

Lam, L.K., V.L. Sparnins, and L.W. Wattenberg. 1982. "Isolation and Identification of Kahweol Palmitate and Cafestol Palmitate as Active Constituents of Green Coffee Beans that Enhance Glutathione S-Transferase Activity in the Mouse." *Cancer Research* 42, no. 4, pp. 1193–98.

Leidy, H.J., P.M. Clifton, A. Astrup, T.P. Wycherley, M.S. Westerterp-Plantenga, N.D. Luscombe-Marsh, S.C. Woods, and R.D. Mattes. 2015. "The Role of Protein in Weight Loss and Maintenance." *American Journal of Clinical Nutrition*, pp. 1320S–29S. doi:10.3945/ajcn.114.084038

Márquez, F., N. Babio, M. Bulló, and J. Salas-Salvadó. 2012. "Evaluation of the Safety and Efficacy of Hydroxycitric Acid or Garcinia Cambogia Extracts in Humans." *Critical Reviews in Food Science and Nutrition* 52, no. 7, pp. 585–94. doi:10.1080/10408398.2010.500551

Martin, W.F., L.E. Armstrong, and N.R. Rodriguez. 2005. "Dietary Protein Intake and Renal Function." *Nutrition & Metabolism* 2, no. 1, p. 25. doi:10.1186/1743-7075-2-25

Mattes, R.D., and L. Bormann. 2000. "Effects of (-)-Hydroxycitric Acid on Appetitive Variables." *Physiology & Behavior* 71, no. 1–2, pp. 87–94. doi:10.1016/s0031-9384(00)00321-8

Motil, K.J., D.E. Matthews, D.M. Bier, J.F. Burke, H.N. Munro, and V.R. Young. 1981. "Whole-Body Leucine and Lysine Metabolism: Response to Dietary Protein Intake in Young Men." *American Journal of Physiology-Endocrinology and Metabolism* 240, no. 6, pp. E712–21.

Murray, R. 1987. "The Effects of Consuming Carbohydrate-Electrolyte Beverages on Gastric Emptying and Fluid Absorption During and Following Exercise." *Sports Medicine* 4, no. 5, pp. 322–51. doi:10.2165/00007256-198704050-00002

Murray, R. 1995. "Fluid Needs in Hot and Cold Environments." *Internal Journal of Sports Nutrition* 5, pp. S62–S73.

Natural Medicines. 2015. https://naturalmedicines.therapeuticresearch.com/

Ogden, C.L., M.D. Carroll, B.K. Kit, and K.M. Flegal. 2012. "Prevalence of Obesity and Trends in Body Mass Index Among US Children and Adolescents, 1999–2010." *JAMA: The Journal of the American Medical Association* 307, no. 5, pp. 483–90. doi:10.1001/jama.2012.40

Onakpoya, I., R. Terry, and E. Ernst. 2011. "The Use of Green Coffee Extract as a Weight Loss Supplement: A Systematic Review and Meta-Analysis of Randomised Clinical Trials." *Gastroenterology Research and Practice* 2011, pp. 1–6. doi:10.1155/2011/382852

Onakpoya, I., S.K. Hung, R. Perry, B. Wider, and E. Ernst. 2011. "The Use of Garcinia Extract (Hydroxycitric Acid) as a Weight Loss Supplement: A Systematic Review and Meta-Analysis of Randomised Clinical Trials." *Journal of Obesity* 2011, pp. 1–9: 509038. doi:10.1155/2011/509038

Passe, D.H., M. Horn, and R. Murray. 1997. "The Effects of Beverage Carbonation on Sensory Responses and Voluntary Fluid intake Following Exercise." *International Journal of Sports Nutrition* 7, no. 4, pp. 286–97.

Pinchan, G., R.K. Gauttam, O.S. Tomar, and A.C. Bajaj. 1988. "Effects of Primary Hypohydration of Physical Work Capacity." *International Journal of Biometeorology* 32, no. 3, pp. 176–80. doi:10.1007/bf01045276

Rabito, M.J., and A.D. Kaye. 2013. "Complementary and Alternative Medicine and Cardiovascular Disease: An Evidence-Based Review." *Evidence-Based Complementary and Alternative Medicine* 2013, pp. 1–8: 672097. doi:10.1155/2013/672097.

Ramalakshmi, K., I.R. Kubra, and L.J. Rao. 2007. "Physicochemical Characterisitics of Green Coffee: Comparison of Graded and Defective Beans." *Journal of Food Science* 72, no. 5, pp. S333–37. doi:10.1111/j.1750-3841.2007.00379.x

Ribeiro, J.A., and A.M. Sebastião. 2010. "Caffeine and Adenosine." *Journal of Alzheimers Disease:JAD*, pp. S3–15.

Roman, R.R., S.J. Flores, and A. Alarcon. 1996. "Control of Obesity with Garcinia Cambogia Extract." *Investigacion Medica Internacional* 22, pp. 97–100.

Sawka, M.N., and E.F. Coyle. 1999. "Influence of Body Water and Blood Volume on Thermoregulation and Exercise Performance in the Heat." *Exercise and Sport Sciences Reviews* 27, pp. 167–218. doi:10.1249/00003677-199900270-00008

Sawka, M.N., L.M. Burke, E.R. Eichner, R.J. Maughan, S.J. Montain, and N.S. Stachenfeld. 2007. "American College of Sports Medicine Position Stand. Exercise and Fluid Replacement." *Medicine and Science in Sports and Exercise* 39, no. 2, pp. 377–90.

Sawka, M.N., A.J. Young, R.P. Francesconi, S.R. Muza, and K.B. Pandolf. 1985. "Thermoregulatory and Blood Responses During Exercise at Graded Hypohydration Levels." *Journal of Applied Physiology* 59, no. 5, pp. 1394–401.

Semwal, R.B., D.K. Semwal, I. Vermaak, and A. Viljoen. 2015. "A Comprehensive Scientific Overview of Garcinia Cambogia." *Fitoterapia* 102, pp. 134–48. doi:10.1016/j.fitote.2015.02.012

Smith, N., and A.L. Atroch. 2010. "Guaraná's Journey from Regional Tonic to Aphrodisiac and Global Energy Drink." *Evidence-Based Complementary and Alternative Medicine* 7, no. 3, pp. 279–82. doi:10.1093/ecam/nem162

Sorkin, B.C., K.M. Camp, C.J. Haggans, P.A. Deuster, L. Haverkos, P. Maruvada, E. Witt, and P.M. Coates. 2014. "Executive Summary of NIH Workshop on the Use and Biology of Energy Drinks: Current Knowledge and Critical Gaps." *Nutrition Reviews* 72, no. 1, pp. 1–8. doi:10.1111/nure.12154

Suzuki, A., D. Kagawa, R. Ochiai, I. Tokimitsu, and I. Saito. 2002. "Green Coffee Bean Extract and Its Metabolites Have a Hypotensive Effect in Spontaneously Hypertensive Rats." *Hypertension Research* 25, no. 1, pp. 99–107. doi:10.1291/hypres.25.99

U.S. FDA (Food and Drug Administration). 2007. "Medicines in Your Home: Caffeine and Your Body." FDA.Gov. www.fda.gov/downloads/UCM200805. pdf (accessed August 2015).

van Loon, L.J., J.J. van Rooijen, B. Niesen, H. Verhagen, W.H. Saris, and A.J. Wagenmakers. 2000. "Effects of Acute (-)-Hydroxycitrate Supplementation on Substrate Metabolism at Rest and During Exercise in Humans." *The American Journal of Clinical Nutrition* 72, no. 6, pp. 1445–50.

Volpi, E., W.W. Campbell, J.T. Dwyer, M.A. Johnson, G.L. Jensen, J.E. Morley, and R.R. Wolfe. 2013. "Is the Optimal Level of Protein Intake for Older Adults Greater Than the Recommended Dietary Allowance." *The Journals of Gerontology Series A: Biological Sciences and Medical Sciences* 68, no. 6, pp. 667–81. doi:10.1093/gerona/gls229

Watson, J.A., and J.M. Lowenstein. 1970. "Citrate and the Conversion of Carbohydrate into Fat. Fatty Acid Synthesis by a Combination of Cytoplasm and Mitochondria." *Journal of Biological Chemistry* 245, no. 22, pp. 5993–6002.

Werner, J. 1993. "Temperature Regulation During Exercise: An Overview." In *Exercise, Heat, and Thermoregulation*, eds. C.V. Gisolfi, D.R. Lamb, and E.R. Nadel, 48–77. Dubuque, IA: Brown and Benchmark.

Westerterp-Plantenga, M.S., and E.M. Kovacs. 2002. "The Effect of (-)-Hydroxycitrate on Energy Intake and Satiety in Overweight Humans." *International Journal of Obesity Relative Metabolic Disorders* 26, pp. 870–72.

Wilk, B., and O. Bar-Or. 1996. "Effect of Drink Flavor and NaCL on Voluntary Drinking and Hydration in Boys Exercising in the Heat." *Journal of Applied Physiology* 80, no. 4, pp. 1112–17.

Wilk, B., S. Kriemler, H. Keller, and O. Bar-Or. 1998. "Consistency in Preventing Voluntary Dehydration in Boys Who Drink a Flavored Carbohydrate-NaCl Beverage During Exercise in the Heat." *International Journal of Sports and Nutrition* 8, no. 1, pp. 1–9.

APPENDIX A

Additional Resources

Office of Dietary Supplements
(https://ods.od.nih.gov/)

The Dietary Supplement Health and Education Act of 1994 (Public Law 103-417, DSHEA), authorized the establishment of the Office of Dietary Supplements (ODS) at the National Institutes of Health (NIH). The ODS was created in 1995 within the Office of Disease Prevention, Office of the Director, NIH.

The mission of ODS is to strengthen knowledge and understanding of dietary supplements by evaluating scientific information, stimulating and supporting research, disseminating research results, and educating the public to foster an enhanced quality of life and health for the U.S. population.

Natural Medicines
(https://naturalmedicines.therapeuticresearch.com/)

Natural Medicines (formerly Natural Standard and Natural Medicines Comprehensive Database) is impartial, not supported by any interest group, professional organization, or product manufacturer. Natural Medicines offers quick access to comprehensive, evidence-based, peer-reviewed information on foods, herbs, supplements, and natural therapies. Database coverage includes efficacy, adverse effects, interactions, pregnancy, lactation, pharmacology, toxicology, dosing, standardization, and products tested by third-party laboratories. Patient handouts are available.

Natural Medicines was founded by healthcare providers and researchers at Therapeutic Research, publisher of the Pharmacist's Letter and Prescriber's Letter.

Council for Responsible Nutrition
(http://www.crnusa.org/)

The Council for Responsible Nutrition (CRN), founded in 1973 and based in Washington, D.C., is the leading trade association representing dietary supplement and functional food manufacturers and ingredient suppliers. CRN companies produce a large portion of the dietary supplements marketed in the United States and globally. CRN member companies manufacture popular national brands as well as the store brands marketed by major supermarkets, drug stores, and discount chains. These products also include those marketed through natural food stores and mainstream direct selling companies. CRN member companies are expected to comply with a host of federal and state regulations governing dietary supplements in the areas of manufacturing, marketing, quality control, and safety. CRN supplier and manufacturer member companies also agree to adhere to additional voluntary guidelines as well as to CRN's Code of Ethics.

American Botanical Council (www.herbalgram.org)

The American Botanical Council is an independent, nonprofit research and education organization dedicated to providing accurate and reliable information for consumers, healthcare practitioners, researchers, educators, industry, and the media. It provides education using science-based and traditional information to promote responsible use of herbal medicine.

Examine.com (www.Examine.com)

Examine.com is an independent and unbiased encyclopedia on supplementation and nutrition. Examine.com does not accept donations, third-party funding, or sponsorship of any kind. Founded in early 2011, they have one goal—"to be the unbiased source for supplements and nutrition."

Dietary Supplement Intake Assessment: Questions to Ask Clients

The following is a relatively short but effective list of questions to find out what dietary supplements your clients may be using and why and how they use them. The goal is not to imply judgment when inquiring about an individual's choices to use or not to use dietary supplements. Often times, people feel that others do not understand why they would take dietary supplements and would advise them to stop if they were to divulge that they did use them. If you are a health care professional or are seen as an authority in such matters, it is important that the individuals that you counsel trust you and feel that you are objective in your assessment of dietary supplements and their choice to use them. If this trust can be established, you will be able to guide those who are determined to use them toward safe and efficacious options. Without that trust, they will either not disclose their use of supplements or not heed the advice that you provide them about the use of dietary supplements, ultimately leaving them to seek information from the Internet and other profit-oriented media.

Ask each of the following initial questions:

- Do you take any dietary supplements?
- Do you take any herbal products?
- Are there any products you take in the hope of avoiding the need to take medicines?

If the answer is yes to any of the preceding, follow with:

- Why did you first decide to try this product?

- Do you feel you have received any benefit from taking this product?
- How long have you been taking this product?
- How often do you take this product?
- Do you follow the directions on the label of this product?
  - If not, how much of this product do you take?
- Do you plan to continue using this product?
- Do you feel that you have a good understanding of what the ingredients are and how they are supposed to work?
- Do you take any prescription or over-the-counter medications?
- Have you shared with your doctor your decision to use this product?
- Do you feel that this product has ever caused any adverse reaction such as an upset stomach, shakiness, drowsiness, anxiety, headache, hives, or other allergic reaction?

The answers to the previous questions will put you in a position to objectively assess the individual's understanding of dietary supplements and their motivation for using them.

Index

OTHER TITLES IN OUR NUTRITION AND DIETETICS PRACTICE COLLECTION

Katie Ferraro, University of San Francisco School of Nursing, Editor

Nutrition Support
by Brenda O'Day

*Diet and Disease: Nutrition for Heart Disease,
Diabetes, and Metabolic Stress*
by Katie Ferraro

*Diet and Disease: Nutrition for Gastrointestinal, Musculoskeletal,
Hepatobiliary, Pancreatic, and Kidney Diseases*
by Katie Ferraro

Weight Management and Obesity
by Courtney Winston Paolicelli

FORTHCOMING TITLES FOR THIS COLLECTION

Introduction to Dietetic Practice
by Katie Ferraro

Sports Nutrition
by Kary Woodruff

Momentum Press is one of the leading book publishers in the field of engineering, mathematics, health, and applied sciences. Momentum Press offers over 30 collections, including Aerospace, Biomedical, Civil, Environmental, Nanomaterials, Geotechnical, and many others.

Momentum Press is actively seeking collection editors as well as authors. For more information about becoming an MP author or collection editor, please visit http://www.momentumpress.net/contact

Announcing Digital Content Crafted by Librarians

Momentum Press offers digital content as authoritative treatments of advanced engineering topics by leaders in their field. Hosted on ebrary, MP provides practitioners, researchers, faculty, and students in engineering, science, and industry with innovative electronic content in sensors and controls engineering, advanced energy engineering, manufacturing, and materials science.

Momentum Press offers library-friendly terms:

- perpetual access for a one-time fee
- no subscriptions or access fees required
- unlimited concurrent usage permitted
- downloadable PDFs provided
- free MARC records included
- free trials

The **Momentum Press** digital library is very affordable, with no obligation to buy in future years.

For more information, please visit **www.momentumpress.net/library** or to set up a trial in the US, please contact **mpsales@globalepress.com**.

CPSIA information can be obtained
at www.ICGtesting.com
Printed in the USA
FSHW020025221120
76019FS

9 781606 507551